Summary

Update: On June 20, 2012, the House of Representatives passed, by voice vote and under suspension of the rules, S. 3187 (EAH), the Food and Drug Administration Safety and Innovation Act, as amended. This bill would reauthorize the FDA prescription drug and medical device user fee programs (which would otherwise expire on September 30, 2012), create new user fee programs for generic and biosimilar drug approvals, and make other revisions to other FDA drug and device approval processes. It reflects bicameral compromise on earlier versions of the bill (S. 3187 [ES], which passed the Senate on May 24, 2012, and H.R. 5651 [EH], which passed the House on May 30, 2012). The following CRS reports provide overview information on FDA's processes for approval and regulation of drugs:

- CRS Report R41983, *How FDA Approves Drugs and Regulates Their Safety and Effectiveness*, by Susan Thaul.

- CRS Report RL33986, *FDA's Authority to Ensure That Drugs Prescribed to Children Are Safe and Effective*, by Susan Thaul.

- CRS Report R42130, *FDA Regulation of Medical Devices*, by Judith A. Johnson.

- CRS Report R42508, *The FDA Medical Device User Fee Program*, by Judith A. Johnson.

(Note: The rest of this report has not been updated since April 24, 2012.)

The Food and Drug Administration (FDA) is the agency responsible for the regulation of medical devices. These are a wide range of products that are used to diagnose, treat, monitor, or prevent a disease or condition in a patient. A company must obtain FDA's prior approval or clearance before marketing many medical devices in the United States. The Center for Devices and Radiological Health (CDRH) within FDA is primarily responsible for medical device review and regulation.

Congress first gave FDA the authority to collect user fees from medical device companies in the Medical Device User Fee and Modernization Act of 2002 (P.L. 107-250). The purpose of the user fee program is to help reduce the time in which FDA can review and make decisions on marketing applications. Lengthy review times affect the industry, which waits to market its products, and patients, who wait to use these products. The user fee law provides a revenue stream for FDA; in conjunction, the agency negotiates with industry to set *performance goals* for the premarket review of medical devices. Reauthorization of FDA's medical device user fees last occurred in 2007, just before the FDA's authority would expire, via the Medical Device User Fee Amendments of 2007 (MDUFA II). Current authority will expire on October 1, 2012.

On February 1, 2012, FDA announced that it had reached "an agreement in principle" with the medical device industry on proposed recommendations for the second reauthorization—referred to as MDUFA III. A draft MDUFA III package, composed of statutory language and the FDA-industry agreement on performance goals and procedures, was posted on the FDA website on March 14, 2012, and a public meeting describing the draft was held on March 28, 2012. The 30-day comment period on the draft ended April 16, 2012. Following review of the comments, FDA may revise the recommendation and then is to submit the final package to Congress.

Since medical device user fees were first collected in FY2003, they have comprised an increasing proportion of FDA's device budget. Medical device user fees have raised a number of concerns, prompting Congress to carefully consider issues such as which agency activities could use fees, how user fees can be kept from supplanting federal funding, and which companies should qualify as a small business and pay a reduced fee.

Congress is also considering reauthorization of the Prescription Drug User Fee Act (PDUFA) as well as new proposals for a Generic Drug User Fee Act and a Biosimilars User Fee Act. It is likely that these three will be combined with MDUFA III along with a variety of related and unrelated issues. Because of the importance of user fees to FDA's budget, PDUFA and MDUFA are considered to be "must pass" legislation, and Congress has often in the past included language to address a range of other concerns. For example, MDUFA II included provisions about the extent to which FDA can delegate activities to third parties, a unique device identification system, and reporting requirements for devices linked to serious injuries or deaths. House and Senate committees are circulating discussion drafts that contain many proposals that would affect medical device regulation. FDA has indicated that some of these pending reforms could conflict with what was negotiated with industry in the MDUFA III proposal. Some reforms are of concern because they would require more agency resources; others were discussed during the user fee negotiations and were set aside. If MDUFA reauthorization does not occur by early summer, federal regulations require that reduction-in-force notices be sent out in July 2012, giving 60 days' advance notice to about 250 FDA employees that their employment under the MDUFA program would end September 30, 2012.

Contents

Figures

Tables

Appendixes

Contacts

Introduction

Update: On June 20, 2012, the House of Representatives passed, by voice vote and under suspension of the rules, S. 3187 (EAH), the Food and Drug Administration Safety and Innovation Act, as amended. This bill would reauthorize the FDA prescription drug and medical device user fee programs (which would otherwise expire on September 30, 2012), create new user fee programs for generic and biosimilar drug approvals, and make other revisions to other FDA drug and device approval processes. It reflects bicameral compromise on earlier versions of the bill (S. 3187 [ES], which passed the Senate on May 24, 2012, and HR 5651 [EH], which passed the House on May 30, 2012). The following CRS reports provide overview information on FDA's processes for approval and regulation of drugs:

- CRS Report R41983, *How FDA Approves Drugs and Regulates Their Safety and Effectiveness*, by Susan Thaul.

- CRS Report RL33986, *FDA's Authority to Ensure That Drugs Prescribed to Children Are Safe and Effective*, by Susan Thaul.

- CRS Report R42130, *FDA Regulation of Medical Devices*, by Judith A. Johnson.

- CRS Report R42508, *The FDA Medical Device User Fee Program*, by Judith A. Johnson.

(Note: The rest of this report has not been updated since April 24, 2012.)

In 2002, the Medical Device User Fee and Modernization Act (MDUFMA) gave the Food and Drug Administration (FDA) the authority to collect fees from the medical device industry.[1] User fees and direct appropriations from Congress fund review of medical devices by the FDA. Medical devices are a wide range of products that are used to diagnose, treat, monitor, or prevent a disease or condition in a patient. The Federal Food, Drug and Cosmetic Act (FFDCA) defines a medical device as

> an instrument, apparatus, implement, machine, contrivance, implant, in vitro reagent, or other similar or related article, including any component, part, or accessory, which is (1) recognized in the official National Formulary, or the United States Pharmacopeia, or any supplement to them, (2) intended for use in the diagnosis of disease or other conditions, or in the cure, mitigation, treatment, or prevention of disease, in man or other animals, or (3) intended to affect the structure or any function of the body of man or other animals, and which does not achieve its primary intended purposes through chemical action within or on the body of man or other animals and which is not dependent upon being metabolized for the achievement of its primary intended purposes. (FFDCA §201(h), 21 U.S.C. 301 §201(h))

According to FDA, examples of medical devices "range from simple tongue depressors and bedpans to complex programmable pacemakers with micro-chip technology and laser surgical devices."[2] Medical devices also include in vitro diagnostic products, reagents, test kits, and certain electronic radiation-emitting products with medical applications, such as diagnostic ultrasound products, x-ray machines, and medical lasers.

Manufacturers must obtain FDA approval or clearance before marketing many medical devices in the United States. The Center for Devices and Radiological Health (CDRH) has primary responsibility within FDA for medical device premarket review.[3] The purpose of user fees is to

---

[1] MDUFMA (P.L. 107-250) added Sections 737 and 738 to the Federal Food, Drug and Cosmetic Act (FFDCA) [21 USC 379i and 379j]. MDUFMA was amended twice by the Medical Device Technical Corrections Act of 2004 (MDTCA; P.L. 108-214) and the Medical Device User Fee Stabilization Act of 2005 (MDUFSA; P.L. 109-43).

[2] FDA, Medical Devices, "Is the Product a Medical Device," at http://www.fda.gov/medicaldevices/deviceregulationandguidance/overview/classifyyourdevice/ucm051512.htm.

[3] Another center, the Center for Biologics Evaluation and Research (CBER), regulates devices associated with blood (continued...)

support the FDA's medical device premarket review program and to help reduce the time it takes the agency to review and make decisions on marketing applications. Prior to 2002, multiple government reports, as early as 1983, indicated that FDA had insufficient resources for its medical devices premarket review program.[4] Lengthy review times affect the industry, which waits to market its products, and patients, who wait to use these products. The user fee law provides revenue for FDA; in conjunction, the agency negotiates with industry to set *performance goals* for the premarket review of medical devices. The medical device user fee program was modeled after the Prescription Drug User Fee Act (PDUFA).[5]

Like the prescription drug and animal drug user fee programs, the medical device user fee program has been authorized in five-year increments.[6] FDA's medical device user fee authorities were reauthorized just before their expiration by the Medical Device User Fee Amendments of 2007 (MDUFA).[7] The agency's current authority to collect medical device user fees will expire on October 1, 2012.

On February 1, 2012, FDA announced that it had reached "an agreement in principle" with the medical device industry on proposed recommendations for the reauthorization of the medical device user fee program.[8] Referred to as MDUFA III, a draft of the negotiated package—composed of statutory language and the FDA-industry agreement on performance goals and procedures—was posted on the FDA website on March 14, 2012.[9] A public meeting describing the draft was held on March 28, 2012. The 30-day comment period on the draft ended April 16,

---

(...continued)

collection and processing procedures, cellular products, and tissues. For more information, see CRS Report R42130, *FDA Regulation of Medical Devices*, by Judith A. Johnson.

[4] These reports are listed in Institute of Medicine (IOM), *Medical Devices and the Public's Health The FDA 510(k) Clearance Process at 35 Years*, Washington, DC, July 2011, p. 30, http://www.iom.edu/Reports/2011/Medical-Devices-and-the-Publics-Health-The-FDA-510k-Clearance-Process-at-35-Years.aspx.

[5] PDUFA came about following negotiations among the FDA (under Commissioner David Kessler), the drug industry, and key congressional committee Members and staff. The aim of the negotiations was "getting enough qualified doctors onto the FDA staff to carry out drug reviews, and getting the company staffs to cooperate in meeting higher standards. The solution that emerged was one intended to bypass the anachronistic and unreliable congressional system that always underfinanced the FDA." Phillip J. Hilts, *Protecting America's Health* (New York: Alfred A. Knopf, 2003), p. 278. Other key features of PDUFA include ensuring that the user fee revenue would not go to general funds but could be spent only on the drug review program, a sunset provision ensuring the user fee program would be reevaluated every five years, and "an implicit contract by Congress not to exploit the availability of the user fee monies and then reduce FDA appropriations for drug review-related purposes." Daniel Carpenter, *Reputation and Power Organizational Image and Pharmaceutical Regulation at the FDA* (Princeton, NJ: Princeton University Press, 2010), pp. 459-460.

[6] See CRS Report R42366, *Prescription Drug User Fee Act (PDUFA) Issues for Reauthorization (PDUFA V) in 2012*, by Susan Thaul, and CRS Report RL34459, *Animal Drug User Fee Programs*, by Sarah A. Lister.

[7] MDUFA was enacted as Title II of the Food and Drug Administration Amendments Act of 2007 (FDAAA; P.L. 110-85). See CRS Report RL34465, *FDA Amendments Act of 2007 (P.L. 110-85)*, by Erin D. Williams and Susan Thaul.

[8] Food and Drug Administration, "FDA and Industry reach agreement in principle on medical device user fees," press release, February 1, 2012, http://www.fda.gov/NewsEvents/Newsroom/PressAnnouncements/ucm289828.htm. FDA and industry missed the January 15, 2012, statutory deadline for transmitting the MDUFA III package to Congress, delaying the reauthorization process and possibly jeopardizing completion before the medical device user fee program sunsets on September 30, 2012.

[9] FDA, "Draft MDUFA III Commitment Letter," dated February 17, 2012, and posted on FDA website March 14, 2012, at http://www.fda.gov/downloads/MedicalDevices/NewsEvents/WorkshopsConferences/UCM295454.pdf. Document is referred to, at times, as the Commitment Letter or the Agreement. FDA, draft statutory language dated February 17, 2012, and posted at http://www.fda.gov/downloads/MedicalDevices/NewsEvents/WorkshopsConferences/UCM295424.pdf.

2012. Following review of the comments, FDA may revise the recommendation and then is to submit the final package to Congress.

This report describes current law regarding medical device user fees, the impact of MDUFA on FDA review time of various medical device applications and the agency's medical device program budget, the MDUFA III proposal (legislative language and performance goals agreement), and issues that Congress is likely to take up as it works on the reauthorization of the medical device user fee program. **Appendix E** provides a list of acronyms used in this report.

Current Law

The Medical Device Amendments of 1976 (P.L. 94-295) was the first major legislation passed to address the premarket review of medical devices. User fees to support the FDA's medical device premarket review program were first authorized by Congress in 2002, 10 years after Congress had provided the authority for prescription drug user fees via PDUFA. For prescription drugs, the manufacturer must pay a fee for each new drug application (NDA) that is submitted to FDA for premarket review. In contrast, most medical devices are exempt from premarket review and do not pay a user fee. Premarket review and payment of the associated fee is required for about a third of the medical devices listed with FDA (see **Figure 1**).

Figure 1. Medical Devices Listed with FDA, FY2003-FY2007, by Premarket Review Process

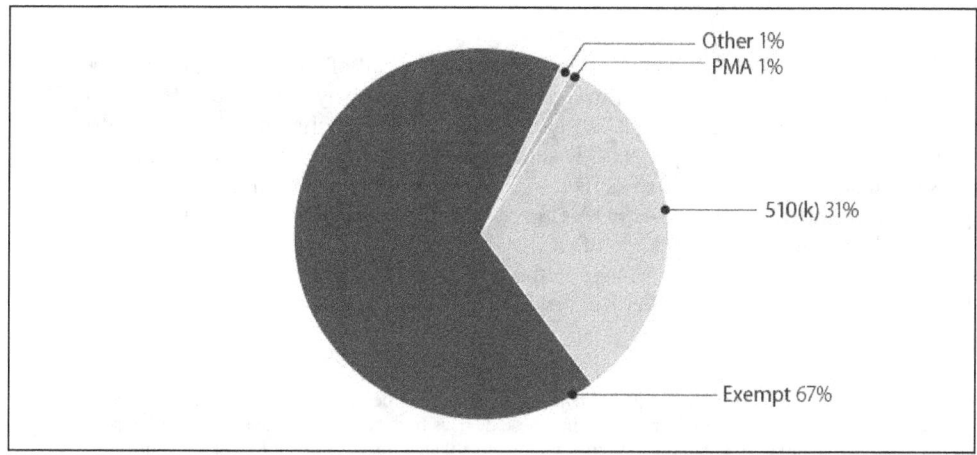

Source: Government Accountabi ity Office, January 2009, GAO-09-190, p. 9.

Notes: "Other" includes devices that were allowed to enter the market via other means, such as through the humanitarian device exemption process that allows market entry, without adherence to certain requirements, for devices benefiting patients with rare diseases or conditions. See "Exemptions and Discounted Fees." Non-exempt devices are reviewed by FDA via the PMA (premarket approval) process or the 510(k) notification. See "FDA Premarket Review of Medical Devices."

FDA Premarket Review of Medical Devices

FDA classifies devices based on the risk to the patient: low-risk devices are Class I, medium-risk are Class II, and high-risk are Class III. Low-risk medical devices (Class I) and a very small number of moderate-risk (Class II) medical devices are exempt from premarket review. In general, for moderate-risk and high-risk medical devices, there are two pathways that manufacturers can use to bring such devices to market with FDA's permission.[10]

One pathway consists of conducting clinical studies, then submitting a premarket approval (PMA) application with evidence providing reasonable assurance that the device is safe and effective. The PMA process is generally used for novel and high-risk devices and is typically lengthy and expensive. It results in a type of FDA permission called *approval*.

Another pathway involves submitting a premarket notification submission—also known as a 510(k), after the section in the FFDCA that authorized this type of notification. With the 510(k), the manufacturer demonstrates that the device is substantially equivalent to a device already on the market (a predicate device) that does not require a PMA. The 510(k) process is unique to medical devices and results in FDA clearance. Substantial equivalence is determined by comparing the performance characteristics of a new device with those of a predicate device.

Medical Device User Fees

Premarket review by FDA—both PMA and 510(k)—requires the payment of a user fee. FDA typically *evaluates* more than 4,000 510(k) notifications and about 40 original PMA applications each year.[11] Since MDUFA II reauthorization in 2007, FDA *cleared* over 13,000 510(k) devices and *approved* 106 PMAs.[12] According to CDRH Director Jeffrey Shuren, for FY2010, user fees collected under MDUFA "fund only about 20% of the device review program"; in contrast, user fees collected under the PDUFA account for over 60% of the drug review program's budget.[13]

There are also fees for when a manufacturer requests approval of a significant change in the design or performance of a device approved via the PMA pathway.[14] This is called a Panel-Track Supplement when it is necessary for FDA to evaluate significant clinical data in order to make a decision on approval of the supplement. If a manufacturer requests approval of a change in aspects of an approved device, such as its design, specifications, or labeling, this is called a 180-Day PMA Supplement. In this case, FDA either does not require new clinical data or requires only limited clinical data. When a manufacturer requests approval for a minor change to an approved device, such as a minor change in the design or labeling, this is called a Real-Time PMA Supplement. With a Premarket Report, a manufacturer requests the approval of a high-risk

---

[10] Novel devices lacking a legally marketed predicate are automatically designated Class III. FFDCA Section 513(f) established an expedited mechanism for reclassifying these devices based on risk, reducing the regulatory burden on manufacturers. The de novo 510(k), though requiring more data than a traditional 510(k), often requires less information than a PMA application. For more information on device classification and the FDA review process, see CRS Report R42130, *FDA Regulation of Medical Devices*, by Judith A. Johnson.

[11] U.S. Congress, Senate Special Committee on Aging, A Delicate Balance: FDA and the Reform of the Medical Device Approval Process, Testimony of William Maisel, Deputy Center Director for Science, FDA/CDRH, 112th Cong., 1st sess., April 13, 2011.

[12] U.S. Congress, House Committee on Energy and Commerce, Subcommittee on Health, *Reauthorization of MDUFA What it means for jobs, innovation and patients*, Statement of Jeffrey Shuren, CDRH Director, FDA, 112th Cong., 2nd sess., February 15, 2012; and U.S. Congress, Senate Committee on Health, Education, Labor and Pensions, *FDA User Fee Agreements*, Statement of Jeffrey Shuren, CDRH Director, FDA, 112th Cong., 2nd sess., March 29, 2012.

[13] Ibid.

[14] FFDCA 738(a)(2)(A).

device, originally approved for single use (one patient, one procedure), for reprocessing to allow additional use.

The original 2002 user fee law had only authorized FDA to collect fees for premarket review, such as for PMA applications or 510(k) notifications. The 2007 reauthorization—MDUFA II—added two new types of annual fees in order to generate a more stable revenue stream for the agency. According to FDA, there were fluctuations in the numbers submitted from year to year, and fee revenues repeatedly fell short of expectations.[15] MDUFA II added *establishment fees*, paid annually by most device establishments registered with FDA, and *product fees*, paid annually for high-risk (Class III) devices for which periodic reporting is required. The annual fees were projected to generate about 50% of the total device fee revenue from FY2008 to FY2012.[16] MDUFA II also added two new application fees, the 30-Day Notice and 513(g) application, and substantially lowered all the existing application fee amounts (see **Table C-1**). A manufacturer uses a 30-Day Notice when requesting to make modifications to manufacturing procedures or methods of manufacture affecting the safety and effectiveness of the device, and a manufacturer requests information on the classification of a device with a 513(g) application.[17]

Other than the establishment fee, the amount of each type of user fee is set as a percentage of the PMA fee, also called the *base fee*. The law prescribes both the base fee amount for each fiscal year, and the percentage of the base fee that constitutes most other fees. For example, the 510(k) fee is equal to 1.84% of the PMA fee. MDUFA II raised the PMA fee by 8.5% per year from FY2008 to FY2012[18] (see **Table C-1**). FDA asserted that this annual increase would ensure that fee revenues contribute their expected share to total program costs, and would provide industry with stability and predictability in the fee revenues it would expect to pay.[19] The amount of the establishment fee (also known as the *establishment registration fee*) was authorized under MDUFA II to rise 8.5% per year from FY2008 to FY2012[20] (see **Table C-1**).

Exemptions and Discounted Fees

Certain types of medical devices, sponsors of medical device PMA applications or 510(k) notifications, and medical device manufacturers are exempt from paying fees, and small businesses pay a reduced rate.[21] Humanitarian Device Exemption (HDE) applications are exempt from user fees, other than establishment fees.[22] An HDE exempts devices that meet certain

---

[15] FDA, "Medical Device User Fee and Modernization Act; Public Meeting," 72 *Federal Register* 19528, April 18, 2007.

[16] FDA, "Medical Device User Fee and Modernization Act; Public Meeting," 72 *Federal Register* 19528, April 18, 2007.

[17] FFDCA 738(a)(2)(A)

[18] FFDCA 738(b).

[19] FDA, "Medical Device User Fee and Modernization Act; Public Meeting," 72 *Federal Register* 19528, April 18, 2007. Under MDUFMA, base fees increased by 34% from FY2003 to FY2004, by 15.7% from FY2004 to FY2005, and by 8.5% from FY2005 to FY2006 and FY2006 to FY2007.

[20] The HHS Secretary had the authority to increase the establishment fee by up to an additional 8.5% (over the annual 8.5% increase) in FY2010 if fewer than 12,250 establishments paid the fee in FY2009. This measure was designed to ensure that the establishment fees were 45% of total fees, ensuring that FDA had a stable funding base from user fees.

[21] FFDCA 738(a)(2)(B); 21 USC 379j(a)(2)(b).

[22] FFDCA 738(a)(2)(B)(i). HDE is intended to encourage the development of devices that aid in the treatment and diagnosis of diseases or conditions that affect fewer than 4,000 individuals in the United States per year. FFDCA 520(m); 21 USC 360j(m). The research and development costs of such devices could exceed the market returns for
(continued...)

---

criteria from the effectiveness requirements of premarket approval. Devices intended solely for pediatric use are exempt from fees other than establishment fees.[23] If an applicant obtains an exemption under this provision, and later submits a supplement for adult use, that supplement is subject to the fee then in effect for an original PMA.

State and federal government entities are exempt from fees for a PMA, premarket report, supplement, 510(k), and establishment registration unless the device is to be distributed commercially. Indian tribes are exempted from having to pay establishment registration fees, unless the device is to be distributed commercially. Other than an establishment fee, the FDA cannot charge a fee for premarket applications for biologics licenses and licenses for biosimilar or interchangeable products if products are licensed exclusively for further manufacturing use.[24]

Under a program authorized by Congress, FDA accredits third parties, allowing them to conduct the initial review of 510(k)s for the purpose of classification of certain devices.[25] The purpose is to improve the efficiency and timeliness of FDA's 510(k) process. No FDA fee is assessed for 510(k) submissions reviewed by accredited third parties, although the third parties charge manufacturers a fee for their services.[26]

In MDUFA II, Congress amended the process of qualifying for small business user fee discounts in response to frustrations expressed by domestic and foreign companies that had difficulties with the requirements. Small businesses—those with gross receipts below a certain amount—pay reduced user fees and have some fees waived altogether.[27] These fee reductions and exemptions are important, because many device companies are small businesses.[28]

Under current law, whether a device company is considered a small business eligible for fee reductions or waivers depends on the particular fee. Small businesses reporting under $30 million in gross receipts or sales are exempt from fees for their first PMA. Proof of receipts may consist of IRS tax documents or qualifying documentation from a foreign government. Companies with annual gross sales or receipts of $100 million or less pay at a rate of 50% of the 510(k) user fee, 30-day notice, request for classification information, and 25% of most other user fees.[29] Small businesses must pay the full amount of the establishment fees.

2007 GAO Study

A March 2007 Government Accountability Office (GAO) report analyzed company revenue information for 50% of the "4,500 device applications subject to user fees that were submitted in FY2006." The remaining 50% of applications "were likely submitted by private companies that did not qualify as small businesses," and GAO was "unable to identify the number of these companies." For the companies that GAO was able to analyze, the report found that 95% of the 697 companies qualifying as small businesses in FY2006 had revenues below $30 million. Of these 697

(...continued)

products that address diseases or conditions affecting small patient populations.

[23] FFDCA 738(a)(2)(B)(v)

[24] FFDCA 738(a)(2)(B)(ii); FFDCA 738(a)(3)(A)

[25] FFDCA 523.

[26] FFDCA 738(a)(2)(B)(iv).

[27] FFDCA 738(d),(e); 21 USC 379j(d),(e).

[28] FDA, "Medical Device User Fee and Modernization Act; Public Meeting," 72 *Federal Register* 19528, April 18, 2007.

[29] FFCCA 738(d); 21 USC 379j(d).

companies, "two-thirds submitted at least one device app ication subject to user fees during that year. These companies were responsible for about 20% of the approximately 4,500 device app ications subject to user fees that were submitted to FDA in FY2006." GAO also analyzed the annual revenue for 258 publicly traded companies that submitted applications subject to user fees and did not qua ify as small businesses in FY2006. Of these 258 companies, 155 (60%) had annual revenue higher than $500 million, 47 companies were above $100 million but at or below $500 million, and 56 companies were at or below the $100 million threshold for small business qualification. GAO did not determine why these companies were not qualified as small businesses. These 258 publicly traded companies were responsible for about 30% of the approximately 4,500 applications subject to user fees submitted to FDA in FY2006.

Source: GAO, "Food and Drug Administration: Revenue Information on Certain Companies Participating in the Medical Device User Fee Program," GAO-07-571R (March 30, 2007), at http://www.gao.gov/assets/100/94743.pdf.

Use of User Fees

A key element of FDA user fee laws—both MDUFA and PDUFA—is that the user fees are to supplement congressional appropriations, not replace them. The law includes complex formulas, called triggers, to enforce that goal. FDA may collect and use MDUFA fees only if the direct appropriations for the activities involved in the premarket review of medical devices and for FDA activities overall remain at a level at least equal (adjusted for inflation) to the pre-MDUFA budget.[30]

Other MDUFA Requirements

Over time, Congress has changed PDUFA to allow user fee revenue to be used for not only FDA activities related to premarket review but also the review of postmarket safety information associated with a drug. In contrast, MDUFA revenue can be used only for activities associated with FDA review of PMAs, 510(k)s, supplements, and reports. The law states that fees "shall only be collected and available to defray increases in the costs of resources allocated for the *process for the review of device applications.*"[31]

MDUFA II added a new Section 738A regarding required reports and outlining the reauthorization process. This section required the Secretary to submit annual fiscal and performance reports for FY2008 through FY2012 to the Senate Committee on Health, Education, Labor, and Pensions, and the House Committee on Energy and Commerce. Fiscal reports address the implementation of FDA's authority to collect medical device user fees, as well as FDA's use of the fees. Performance reports address FDA's progress toward and future plans for achieving the fee-related performance goals identified in the agreement.

The new section also directed the FDA to develop a reauthorization proposal for FY2013 through FY2017 in consultation with specified congressional committees, scientific and academic experts,

---

[30] FFDCA 738(g).

[31] Emphasis added. FFDCA 738(h)(2)(A)(ii). The law specifically defines "costs of resources allocated for the process for the review of device applications" and what activities are considered part of the *"process for the review of device applications."* For example, costs include management of information and activities associated with the process for review include inspections of manufacturing establishments. [Emphasis added. FFDCA 737(8)-(9).] The process for review of device applications focuses solely on activities involved in premarket approval, with one exception: the evaluation of postmarket studies that are required as a condition of approval of certain premarket applications or reports. [FFDCA 737(8)(J).]

health care professionals, patient and consumer advocacy groups, and the regulated industry.[32] Prior to negotiations with industry, FDA was required to request public input, hold a public meeting, and publish public comments on the agency's website. During negotiations with industry, FDA was mandated to hold monthly discussions with patient and consumer advocacy groups to receive their suggestions and discuss their views on the reauthorization. After negotiations with industry were completed, FDA was required to present the recommendations to certain congressional committees, publish the recommendations in the *Federal Register*, provide a 30-day public comment period, hold another public meeting to receive views from stakeholders, and revise the recommendations as necessary. As explained earlier, the FDA missed the new statutory deadline that required the transmittal of the revised recommendations to Congress not later than January 15, 2012.[33] Minutes of all negotiation meetings between FDA and industry were required to be posted on the FDA website.

MDUFA Impact on FDA Review Time and Budget

The amount of time it takes FDA to reach a review decision to clear a 510(k) notification or approve a PMA application are measures of how well the agency is meeting the goals defined in the MDUFA agreement between FDA and the medical device industry. The time it takes to review a medical device—total review time—is composed of the time FDA handles the application— FDA time—plus the amount of time the device sponsor or submitter requires to respond to requests by FDA for additional information about the device.

According to CDRH Director Shuren, "FDA has been meeting or exceeding goals agreed to by FDA and industry under MDUFA II for approximately 95% of the submissions we review each year. For example, FDA completes at least 90% of 510(k) reviews within 90 days or less."[34] However, Dr. Shuren noted that these "metrics reflect FDA time only; they do not reflect the time taken by device sponsors to respond to requests for additional information. Overall time to decision—the time that FDA has the application, plus the time the manufacturer spends answering any questions FDA may have—has increased steadily since 2001."[35]

Figure 2 shows that while the amount of time FDA spends reviewing a 510(k) has decreased, the average total days for the review of 510(k)s has been increasing. FDA and GAO have both studied this issue of increasing review time. A 2011 FDA analysis of the reasons behind the increased average total days for the review of 510(k)s found that FDA reviewers needed to ask for additional information—called an AI Letter—from the 510(k) device manufacturer or sponsor due to the poor quality of the original submission.[36] According to FDA, these quality issues involved "the device description, meaning the sponsor either did not provide sufficient

---

[32] FFDCA 738A(b)

[33] FFDCA 738A(b)(5).

[34] U.S. Congress, House Committee on Energy and Commerce, Subcommittee on Health, *Reauthorization of MDUFA What it means for jobs, innovation and patients*, Statement of Jeffrey Shuren, CDRH Director, FDA, 112th Cong., 2nd sess., February 15, 2012; and, U.S. Congress, Senate Committee on Health, Education, Labor and Pensions, *FDA User Fee Agreements*, Statement of Jeffrey Shuren, CDRH Director, FDA, 112th Cong., 2nd sess., March 29, 2012.

[35] Ibid.

[36] FDA/CDRH, *Analysis of Premarket Review Times Under the 510(k) Program*, July 2011, at http://www.fda.gov/downloads/AboutFDA/CentersOffices/OfficeofMedicalProductsandTobacco/CDRH/CDRHReports/UCM263386.pdf.

information about the device to determine what it was developed to do, or the device description was inconsistent throughout the submission."[37]

Figure 2. Average Time to Decision: 510(k)s

Fiscal Year Receipt Cohorts as of March 11, 2012

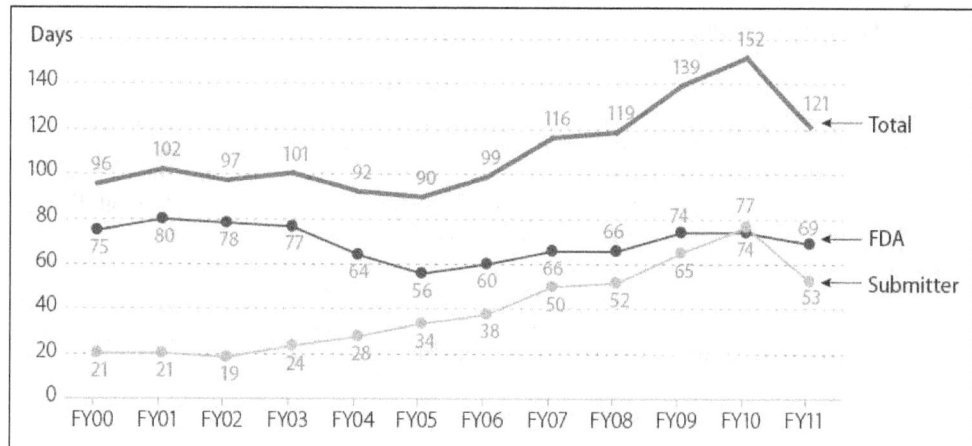

Source: Figure in testimony of CDRH Director Jeffrey Shuren before the Senate HELP Committee, March 29, 2012.

Notes: FDA Days + Submitter Days = Total Time to Decision; times may not add due to rounding. A cohort consists of all 510(k) submissions filed in the same fiscal year. FY2008 through FY2011 cohorts are still open; FY2011 cohort is only 85% closed, and average times will increase.

Furthermore, FDA concluded that "sponsors' failure to address deficiencies identified in first-round AI Letters are major contributors to the increase in total review times. For example, 65% of the time FDA sent a second-round AI Letter because the sponsor failed to submit information requested in the first AI Letter."[38] The 2011 FDA analysis also found "in some cases, the FDA sent AI Letters for inappropriate reasons, such as asking for additional testing that was outside the scope of what would be required for a 510(k) submission, or asking for supporting documentation that was already covered by a standard government form."[39]

---

[37] Ibid., p. 3. Page 15 of the 2011 FDA/CDRH 510(k) report provides more detail on these deficiencies: "(i) the sponsor did not submit required information without justification – such information includes supporting data required under current guidance or performance data that FDA consistently requires for certain device types; (ii) the sponsor failed to identify a predicate; or (iii) the sponsor employed different device descriptions or indications for use for the subject device throughout its submission. In all of these cases, FDA could not reach a substantial equivalence determination without the sponsor providing additional information or rectifying deficiencies in the submission."

[38] Ibid., p. 15.

[39] Ibid., p. 7. Two separate analyses of AI Letters were conducted: one to assess incoming submission quality (Cohort 1) and one to assess the drivers of the increasing numbers of review cycles (Cohort 2). On page 3 of the July 2011 *Analysis of Premarket Review Times Under the 510(k) Program* report, FDA states that it analyzed AI letters "to determine how often the questions that were asked were appropriate or inappropriate, i.e. were the AI Letters justified or did the reviewer ask for information or data that were not permissible as a matter of federal law or FDA policy, or unnecessary to make an SE [substantially equivalent] determination. Results from Cohort 1 showed that reviewers asked for data that had not previously been requested for particular device types 12% of the time. Of those requests, 4% were appropriate, and 8% were inappropriate. Results of the first-round AI Letters from Cohort 2 showed that reviewers asked for appropriate data that had not previously been requested for particular device types 4% of the time, (continued...)

GAO also performed an analysis of FDA performance goals regarding 510(k) device review times and requests for additional information from sponsors.[40] GAO found that although FDA met all medical device performance goals for 510(k)s, the total review time—from submission to final decision—has increased substantially in recent years. Regarding the agency's use of AI Letters, the GAO report notes that "the only alternative to requesting additional information is for FDA to reject the submission."[41] Use of the AI Letter allows the sponsors the opportunity to respond, and although the time to final decision is longer, the application has the opportunity to be approved.

Figure 3 provides information on the amount of time FDA spends reviewing non-expedited PMA applications and Panel-Track Supplements. A device may receive expedited review if it is intended to treat or diagnose a life-threatening condition or irreversibly debilitating disease or condition, and it addresses an unmet need.[42] CDRH Director Shuren notes that although FDA is spending less time reviewing PMA applications, the average total days for the review of PMA applications has been increasing since 2004.[43] The February 2012 GAO report found that for FY2003 through FY2010, FDA met most of the goals for PMAs but fell short on most of the goals for expedited PMAs.[44] The February 2012 GAO report found that FDA review time and time to final decision for both types of PMAs were highly variable but generally increased during this period.[45]

(...continued)

and 2% of the time those requests were inappropriate."

[40] U.S. Government Accountability Office, *Medical Devices FDA Has Met Most Performance Goals but Device Reviews Are Taking Longer*, GAO-12-418, February 2012, http://www.gao.gov/products/GAO-12-418.

[41] Ibid., p. 16.

[42] FDA Guidance, Expedited Review of Premarket Submissions for Devices, February 29, 2008, p. 3, at http://www.fda.gov/downloads/MedicalDevices/DeviceRegulationandGuidance/GuidanceDocuments/ucm089698.pdf.

[43] U.S. Congress, House Committee on Energy and Commerce, Subcommittee on Health, *Reauthorization of MDUFA What it means for jobs, innovation and patients*, Statement of Jeffrey Shuren, CDRH Director, FDA, 112th Cong., 2nd sess., February 15, 2012; and, Senate Committee on Health, Education, Labor and Pensions, *FDA User Fee Agreements*, Statement of Jeffrey Shuren, CDRH Director, FDA, 112th Cong., 2nd sess., March 29, 2012.

[44] Ibid., p. 20.

[45] U.S. Government Accountability Office, *Medical Devices FDA Has Met Most Performance Goals but Device Reviews Are Taking Longer*, GAO-12-418, February 2012, p. 20, http://www.gao.gov/products/GAO-12-418.

Figure 3. Average Time to Decision: PMAs and Panel Track Supplements

(Non-expedited)

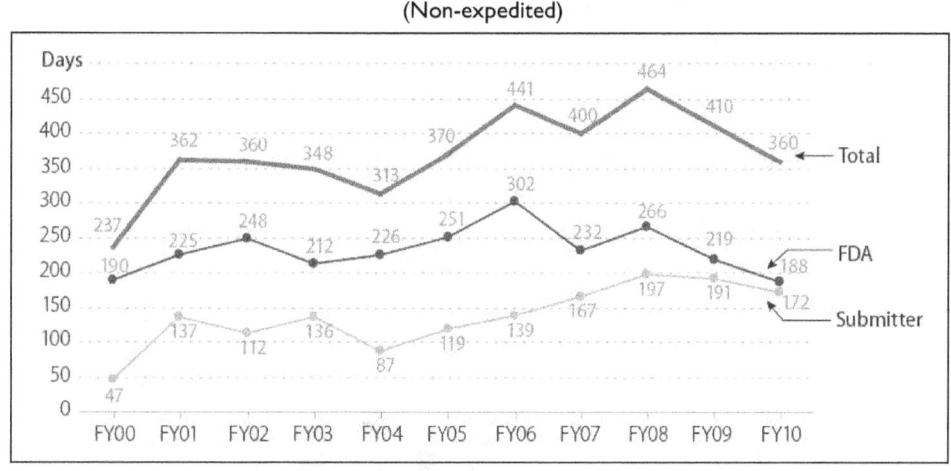

Source: Figure in testimony of CDRH Director Jeffrey Shuren before the Senate HELP Committee, March 29, 2012.

Notes: FDA Days + Submitter Days = Total Time to Decision; times may not add due to rounding. Data is for non-expedited PMAs and Panel-Track Supplements. Some fiscal year cohorts are still open—data may change. A cohort consists of all submissions of a certain type, in this case PMA, filed in the same fiscal year. For FY2010, as of January 30, 2012, there were four applications without a decision; the average time to decision will increase as the cohort closes.

The February 2012 GAO report also commented on communication problems between industry and FDA based on interviews with three industry groups about the medical device review process. These industry representatives noted that FDA "guidance documents are often unclear, out of date, and not comprehensive."[46] They also stated that "after sponsors submit their applications to FDA, insufficient communication from FDA prevents sponsors from learning about deficiencies in their submissions early in FDA's review. According to one of these stakeholders, if FDA communicated these deficiencies earlier in the process, sponsors would be able to correct them and would be less likely to receive a request for additional information."[47] Two industry representatives noted that "review criteria sometimes change after a sponsor submits an application," and one industry representative stated that "criteria sometimes change when the FDA reviewer assigned to the submission changes during the review."[48] The February 2012 GAO report points out that FDA has taken a number of actions to address the issues of the industry representative. For example, FDA has issued new guidance documents, improved the guidance development process, initiated a reviewer certification program for new FDA reviewers, and enhanced its interactive review process for medical devices.

For FY2012, 36% of FDA's total budget comes from user fees.[49] Medical device user fee revenue provides about 10% of the FDA medical device and radiological health program budget.[50] **Figure**

---

[46] Ibid., p. 34.

[47] Ibid.

[48] Ibid., p. 35.

[49] In addition to medical device user fees, Congress has authorized user fees for prescription drugs, animal drugs, animal generic drugs, tobacco products, mammography, color and export certification, and, most recently, several food-related programs.

4 presents the total program level for FDA's device and radiological health program for FY2002 through FY2013 with dollars adjusted for inflation (based on 2005 dollars). **Figure 4** also shows the contribution of medical device user fees, which began in FY2003, to the device and radiological health program budget, as well as fees collected for the inspection of mammography facilities under the Mammography Quality Standards Act (MQSA), which began fee collection in FY1996. For FY2010, user fees collected under MDUFA funded about 20% of the device review program, while user fees collected under PDUFA funded over 60% of the drug review program.

Figure 4. Devices and Radiological Health Program Budget, by Funding Source, for FY2002 to FY2013

(Adjusted to 2005 dollars)

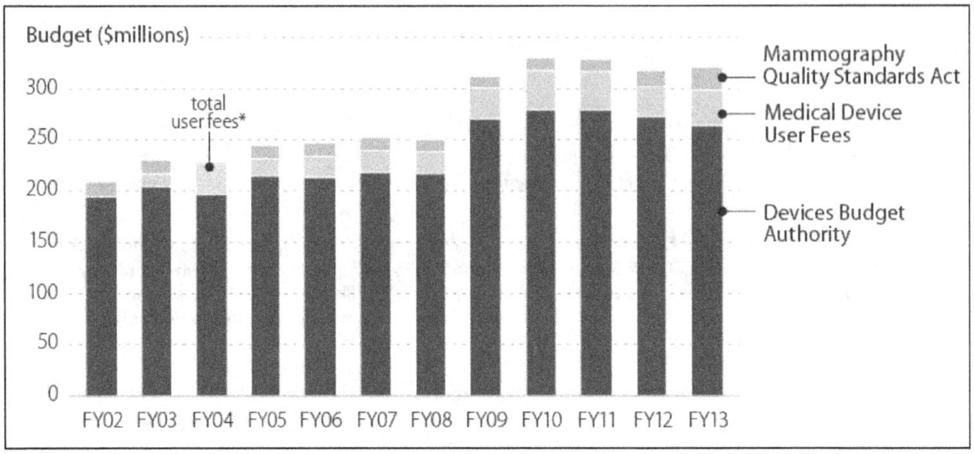

Source: FDA *Justification of Estimates for Appropriations Committees* documents, FY2004 through FY2013.

*Only total user fees were available for FY2004; amounts for medical device user fees and MQSA fees were not identified in the FY2006 *Justification of Estimates for Appropriations Committees*. See **Table 1**.

Notes: Total Program Level = Budget Authority + Medical Device User Fees + MQSA Fees. Data have been adjusted to constant 2005 dollars using "Total Non-Defense" deflators from Office of Management and Budget, *Fiscal Year 2013 Historical Tables, Budget of the U.S. Government*, "Table 10.1, Gross Domestic Product and Deflators Used in the Historical Tables: 1940-2017," pp. 211-212.

User fees are an increasing proportion of FDA's device-related budget, as shown in **Table 1**. User fees were 7.1% of FDA's devices and radiological health program level budget in FY2002 when MQSA was the sole user fee, and 14.2% of FDA's devices and radiological health program level budget in FY2012, with both MQSA and medical device user fees being collected by the agency. **Table 1** shows that over the period of FY2003 to FY2012, the amount of user fees more than doubled, while the amount of direct appropriations (budget authority) increased at a slower rate.

(...continued)

[50] Of the $57.6 million in medical device user fees for FY2012, 60% goes to the devices and radiological health program (funding 221 full-time equivalent employees [FTEs]), 20% to the biologics program (29 FTEs), and the remaining 20% to rent and FDA headquarters (21 FTEs). Data from Department of Health and Human Services (HHS), *Fiscal Year 2013 Food and Drug Administration Justification of Estimates for Appropriations Committees*, February 2012, p. 94.

Table 1. FDA Devices and Radiological Health Program, Fees as a Percentage of Total Program Level

(Unadjusted dollars in millions)

Fiscal Year	Budget Authority	MDUFA[a] Fees	MQSA[b] and Other Fees[c]	Total Fees	Total Fees as % of Total Program Level	Total Program Level
2002	$180.0	$0	$13.7	$13.7	7.1%	$193.7
2003	$193.4	$11.1	$12.9	$24.0	11.0%	$217.3
2004[d]	$191.1	na	na	$30.4	13.7%	$221.5
2005	$215.0	$16.4	$13.0	$29.3	12.0%	$244.3
2006	$220.6	$20.7	$13.8	$34.5	13.5%	$255.0
2007	$230.7	$23.3	$13.6	$36.9	13.8%	$267.5
2008	$237.7	$24.3	$13.3	$37.6	13.7%	$275.3
2009	$298.5	$33.3	$13.5	$46.8	13.6%	$345.3
2010	$313.5	$42.7	$13.8	$56.5	15.3%	$370.0
2011	$322.2	$42.0	$14.4	$56.3	14.9%	$378.5
2012	$322.7	$34.2	$19.1	$53.3	14.2%	$376.0
2013	$319.1	$41.4	$26.3	$67.6	17.5%	$386.8

Source: FDA Justification of Estimates for Appropriations Committees documents, FY2004 through FY2013,

a. MDUFA is Medical Device User Fee Act.

b. MQSA is Mammography Quality Standards Act.

c. For FY2013, the Obama Administration proposes a new Field Reinspection fee and a new International Courier User Fee.

d. The FY2006 *Justification* organized data, including Actual data for FY2004, in a format different than other *Justification* documents (it included rent but did not include the Office of Regulatory Affairs). The FY2007 and FY2008 *Justification* documents provided data in consistent format (without rent but included ORA) for FY2004 Budget Authority, Total Fees, and Total Program Level, but did not provide medical device user fees or MQSA amounts. The FY2006 *Justification* provided the following amounts for Actual FY2004 user fees: medical device user fees, $18.245 million; MQSA, $4.039 million; ORA user fees, $9.071 million.

MDUFA III Proposal

An initial public meeting on the reauthorization of the medical device user fees was held by FDA on September 14, 2010, after which the negotiation process between FDA and industry began, as well as monthly meetings with other stakeholders.[51] Minutes of the 35 negotiation meetings between FDA and the medical device industry are posted on the agency's website, as are minutes

---

[51] FDA, Public Workshop: Medical Device User Fee Program Public Meeting, September 14, 2010, at http://www.fda.gov/MedicalDevices/NewsEvents/WorkshopsConferences/ucm218250.htm.

of the 14 monthly meetings with the other stakeholders, such as health care professional associations and patient and consumer advocacy groups.[52]

On February 1, 2012, FDA announced that it had reached "an agreement in principle on proposed recommendations for the third reauthorization of a medical device user fee program."[53] According to a press release on the FDA website, the recommendations would authorize $595 million in user fees collected by the agency from the medical device industry over a five-year period.[54] FDA would be able to hire more than 200 full-time-equivalent workers with this additional funding. In the minutes for the January 31, 2012, negotiation meeting, industry noted "that MDUFA III represents a sizeable increase of 240 FTEs from current levels, FDA should not expect this type of significant resource increase under MDUFA IV."[55] In response, the agency stated that it had "some concerns about how solid a financial footing this agreement establishes, given that there are a lot of uncertainties about how much effort will be required to meet the goals, and that in order to bring the proposal to a level that Industry could agree to, FDA had to take away any margin of error."[56]

On March 14, 2012, the agency posted on its website the draft negotiated package—composed of statutory language and the FDA-industry agreement on performance goals and procedures— referred to as MDUFA III.[57] A public meeting describing the draft was held on March 28, 2012. The 30-day comment period on the draft ended April 16, 2012. Following review of the comments, FDA may revise the recommendation and then is to submit the final package to Congress.

Update: On June 20, 2012, the House of Representatives passed, by voice vote and under suspension of the rules, S. 3187 (EAH), the Food and Drug Administration Safety and Innovation Act, as amended. This bill would reauthorize the FDA prescription drug and medical device user fee programs (which would otherwise expire on September 30, 2012), create new user fee programs for generic and biosimilar drug approvals, and make other revisions to other FDA drug and device approval processes. It reflects bicameral compromise on earlier versions of the bill (S. 3187 [ES], which passed the Senate on May 24, 2012, and HR 5651 [EH], which passed the House on May 30, 2012). The following CRS reports provide overview information on FDA's processes for approval and regulation of drugs:

- CRS Report R41983, *How FDA Approves Drugs and Regulates Their Safety and Effectiveness*, by Susan Thaul.

- CRS Report RL33986, *FDA's Authority to Ensure That Drugs Prescribed to Children Are Safe and Effective*, by Susan Thaul.

- CRS Report R42130, *FDA Regulation of Medical Devices*, by Judith A. Johnson.

---

[52] FDA, Medical Devices, MDUFA Meetings at http://www.fda.gov/MedicalDevices/DeviceRegulationandGuidance/Overview/MedicalDeviceUserFeeandModernizationActMDUFMA/ucm236902.htm.

[53] Food and Drug Administration, "FDA and Industry reach agreement in principle on medical device user fees," press release, February 1, 2012, http://www.fda.gov/NewsEvents/Newsroom/PressAnnouncements/ucm289828.htm.

[54] Ibid.

[55] FDA, Minutes From Negotiation Meeting on MDUFA III Reauthorization, January 31, 2012, at http://www.fda.gov/MedicalDevices/DeviceRegulationandGuidance/Overview/MedicalDeviceUserFeeandModernizationActMDUFMA/ucm289824.htm.

[56] Ibid.

[57] FDA, draft statutory language dated February 17, 2012, and posted at http://www.fda.gov/downloads/MedicalDevices/NewsEvents/WorkshopsConferences/UCM295424.pdf . FDA, "Draft MDUFA III Commitment Letter," dated February 17, 2012, and posted on FDA website March 14, 2012, at http://www.fda.gov/downloads/MedicalDevices/NewsEvents/WorkshopsConferences/UCM295454.pdf. Document is referred to, at times, as the Commitment Letter or the Agreement.

> • CRS Report R42508, *The FDA Medical Device User Fee Program*, by Judith A. Johnson.
>
> (Note: The rest of this report has not been updated since April 24, 2012.)

Tables in the appendixes provide additional details on the draft MDUFA III proposal beyond the narrative discussion found below. The tables in **Appendix A** relate to the legislative language and the table in **Appendix B** relates to the FDA-industry agreement on performance goals and procedures.

Draft Legislative Language

The draft legislative language portion of the MDUFA III proposal would change the definition of "establishment subject to a registration fee," increasing the number of establishments paying the fee from 16,000 to about 22,000.[58] It would set the fee amount for a PMA in FY2013 at $248,000. The fee amount for a PMA would gradually rise to $268,443 for FY2017. The establishment fee would be $2,575 in FY2013 and rise to $3,872 for FY2016 and FY2017. Other than the establishment fee, the amount of each type of user fee is set as a percentage of the PMA fee, also called the base fee. The draft proposal would keep the percentages the same as in current law except for the 510(k) fee, which would change from 1.84% of the PMA fee to 2% of the PMA fee. Total fee revenue would be set at $97,722,301 for FY2013 and rise to $130,184,348 for FY2017. The total fees collected over the five-year period FY2013 through FY2017 would be $595 million.

The draft MDUFA III legislative language would adjust the total revenue amounts by a specified inflation adjustment, similar to the adjustment made under PDUFA, and the base fee amount would be adjusted as needed on a uniform proportional basis to generate the inflation-adjusted total revenue amount. After the base fee amounts are adjusted for inflation, the establishment fee amount would be further adjusted as necessary so that the total fee collections for the fiscal year would generate the total adjusted revenue amount. The new adjusted fee amounts would be published in the *Federal Register* 60 days before the start of each fiscal year along with the rationale for adjusting the fee amounts.

The draft legislative language includes a provision that would allow FDA to grant a waiver or reduce fees for a PMA or establishment fee "if the waiver is in the interest of public health." According to the FDA presentation at the March 28, 2012, public meeting, the fee waiver is intended for laboratory developed test (LDT) manufacturers. This provision would sunset at the end of MDUFA III.

The draft proposal includes a requirement that sponsors submit an electronic copy of a PMA, 510(k), and other specified submissions and any supplements to such submissions. The requirement would begin after the issuance of final guidance. The draft legislative language also includes a provision for streamlined hiring of FDA employees. The authority for streamlined hiring would terminate three years after enactment.

---

[58] FDA, MDUFA Reauthorization Public Meeting, March 28, 2012.

Draft Industry-FDA Performance Goals and Procedures for MDUFA III: The Agreement

The agreement begins by stating, "FDA and the industry are committed to protecting and promoting public health by providing timely access to safe and effective medical devices. Nothing in this letter precludes the Agency from protecting the public health by exercising its authority to provide a reasonable assurance of the safety and effectiveness of medical devices."[59] The agreement subsequently describes a number of process improvements that aim to improve FDA's medical device review process, provides revised performance goals and new shared outcome goals, describes infrastructure improvements, and provides for an independent assessment of the device review process.

Process Improvements. In comparison to MDUFA II, the discussion of these topics is greatly expanded and consolidated into one new section of the agreement. FDA will put in place a structured process for managing pre-submissions, providing feedback to applicants via e-mail and a one-hour meeting or teleconference. It will publish guidance on electronic submissions and will clarify submission acceptance criteria. The agency will continue to use interactive review to encourage informal communication with the applicant to facilitate timely completion of the review process. FDA will continue to apply user fees to the guidance document development process, and may apply user fees to delete outdated guidance, note which are under review, and provide a list of prioritized device guidance documents intended to be published within a year. It will work with interested parties to improve the current third-party review program. FDA will implement final guidance on factors to consider when making benefit-risk determinations in device premarket review, including patient tolerance for risk and magnitude of benefit. The agency will propose additional low-risk medical devices to exempt from the 510(k) process. FDA will work with industry to develop a transitional in vitro diagnostics (IVD) approach for the regulation of emerging diagnostics.

Review Performance Goals. The main focus of the agreement is FDA's commitment to completing the review of the various medical device submissions—such as PMA reviews and 510(k) notifications—within specified timeframes in exchange for an industry fee to support the review activity. Performance goals are specified for each type of submission and for FY2013 through FY2017; each goal specifies the percentage of applications FDA will complete along with a given time period. See **Table B-1** and **Table D-1** for further details.

Shared Outcome Goals. This is a new section and was not part of the MDUFA II agreement. The purpose of the programs and initiatives outlined in the agreement is to reduce the average total time to decision for PMAs and 510(k)s. FDA and applicants share the responsibility for achieving this goal. For PMA submissions received beginning in FY2013, the average total time to decision goal for FDA and industry is 395 calendar days; beginning in FY2015, 390 calendar days; and beginning in FY2017, 385 calendar days. For 510(k) submissions received beginning in FY2013, the average total time to decision goal for FDA and industry is 135 calendar days; beginning in FY2015, 130 calendar days; and beginning in FY2017, 124 calendar days.

---

[59] FDA, "Draft MDUFA III Commitment Letter," dated February 17, 2012, and posted on FDA website March 14, 2012, at http://www.fda.gov/downloads/MedicalDevices/NewsEvents/WorkshopsConferences/UCM295454.pdf.

Infrastructure. User fees will be used to "reduce the ratio of review staff to front line supervisors in the Pre-market review program."[60] FDA will enhance and supplement scientific review capacity by hiring reviewers and using external experts to assist with device application review. FDA will seek to obtain streamlined hiring authority and work with industry to benchmark best practices for employee retention via financial and non-financial means. User fees will supplement (1) management training; (2) MDUFA III training for all staff; (3) Reviewer Certification Program for new CDRH reviewers; and (4) specialized training to provide continuous learning for all staff. FDA will improve its IT system to allow real-time status information on submissions.

Independent Assessment of Review Process Management. By the end of the second quarter of FY2013, FDA will hire a consultant to assess the device application review process. Within six months of award of the contract, a report on recommendations likely to have a significant impact on review time will be published. The final report will be published within one year of contract award date. FDA will publish a corrective action and implementation plan within six months of receipt of each report. The consultant will evaluate FDA's implementation and publish a report no later than February 1, 2016.

Performance Reports. As was the case in MDUFA II, FDA will meet with industry on a quarterly basis to present data and discuss progress in meeting goals. The agreement requires more detailed information to be covered in quarterly reports by CDRH and CBER; specifically, elements to be included are listed for 510(k)s, PMAs, Pre-Submissions, and Investigational Device Exemptions (IDEs).[61] CDRH reports quarterly and CBER reports annually on 11 additional data points. FDA reports annually on nine other topics.

Discretionary Waiver. FDA will seek authority to grant discretionary fee waivers or reduced fees in the interest of public health. Authority for the waiver and reduced fees would expire at the end of MDUFA III. According to the FDA presentation at the March 28, 2012, public meeting, the fee waiver is intended for laboratory developed test (LDT) manufacturers.

Other Potential Issues

In addition to MDUFA III, Congress is considering reauthorization of PDUFA as well as new proposals for a Generic Drug User Fee Act and a Biosimilars User Fee Act. It is likely that these three will be combined with MDUFA III along with a variety of related and unrelated issues. Because of the importance of user fees to FDA's budget, PDUFA and MDUFA are considered to be "must pass" legislation, and Congress has often in the past included language to address a range of other concerns. For example, MDUFA II included provisions about the extent to which FDA can delegate activities to third parties (inspections and the review of premarket notifications); establishment registration requirements (timing and electronic submission); a unique device identification system; and reporting requirements for devices linked to serious injuries or deaths. Provisions that have been mentioned as possibly being included in current legislation containing FDA user fee authorization include the following:

- reauthorization of Best Pharmaceutical for Children Act (BPCA) and Pediatric Research Equity Act (PREA);

---

[60] Ibid., p. 12.

[61] An IDE allows an unapproved device (most commonly an invasive or life-sustaining device) to be used in a clinical study to collect the data required to support a PMA submission.

- provisions to prevent, avert, or manage drug shortages;

- incentives for antibiotic makers;

- security of the pharmaceutical supply chain;

- less restrictive FDA advisory committee conflict-of-interest waiver policies;

- parity for foreign and domestic manufacturing inspections;

- quicker approval of drugs to treat very rare diseases;

- increased input from patients, hospitals, pharmacists, and others in drug development, review, and postmarket study;

- recall authority for drug products;

- personal-use and commercial drug importation;

- clarification of the least burdensome standard in requesting additional information from sponsors of PMA or 510(k) submissions;

- expanding FDA's authority to require a manufacturer to conduct postmarket surveillance of class II and class III medical devices;

- inclusion of medical devices in the Sentinel Initiative/System;[62]

- extension of the humanitarian device exemption;

- continuation of a demonstration grant program on improving the availability of pediatric devices;

- extension of the third-party review program for 510(k) submissions; and

- limiting the use of a recalled medical device as a predicate in 510(k) submissions.

The House Committee on Energy and Commerce, Subcommittee on Health held a hearing on MDUFA on February 15, 2012, and the Senate Committee on Health, Education, Labor and Pensions held a hearing on FDA user fee agreements on March 29, 2012. The hearing testimony submitted to both the House and Senate by CDRH Director Jeffrey Shuren stated that in FY2010, user fee revenue funded about 20% of the medical device premarket review process; fees collected under MDUFA III would fund about a third of the medical device premarket review process.[63] In contrast, fees collected under PDUFA in FY2010 covered more than 60% of drug review costs. In response to questioning at the Senate hearing, CDRH Director Shuren said if MDUFA reauthorization by Congress has not occurred by early summer, federal regulations require that reduction in force (RIF) notices be sent out in July 2012, giving 60 days' advance notice to about 250 FDA employees that their employment under the MDUFA program would end by September 30, 2012.

---

[62] A national electronic system under development that would transform FDA's ability to track the safety of drugs, biologics, and medical devices once they reach the market. FDA launched the Sentinel Initiative in May 2008; once completed, it would be called the Sentinel System. For more information, see http://www.fda.gov/safety/ FDAsSentinelInitiative/ucm2007250.htm.

[63] U.S. Congress, House Committee on Energy and Commerce, Subcommittee on Health, *Reauthorization of MDUFA What it means for jobs, innovation and patients*, Statement of Jeffrey Shuren, CDRH Director, FDA, 112th Cong., 2nd sess., February 15, 2012; and, U.S. Congress, Senate Committee on Health, Education, Labor and Pensions, *FDA User Fee Agreements*, Statement of Jeffrey Shuren, CDRH Director, FDA, 112th Cong., 2nd sess., March 29, 2012.

The House and Senate committees circulated discussion drafts that contain many of the above listed provisions.[64] CDRH Director Shuren indicated that some of these pending reforms could conflict with what the agency has negotiated with industry in the MDUFA III proposal. "There are several provisions that could have an impact, that could divert resources from implementation of the MDUFA goals and/or that go to issues that were discussed as a part of MDUFA ... that would be counter and would reopen those discussions," according to CDRH Director Shuren.[65] He indicated that proposals regarding device tracking, guidance development, and third-party reviews were of concern, but that "there are many others ... particularly in the House bill."[66] Some proposals are of concern because they would require more agency resources; other proposals were discussed during the user fee negotiations with industry and "taken off the table."[67]

---

[64] The draft Senate bill that contains provisions related to the regulation of medical devices can be found at http://www.help.senate.gov/imo/media/audio/031612_Device_DRAFT_TAM12069.pdf. The draft House bill containing both drug and medical device regulation can be found at http://insidehealthpolicy.com/iwpfile.html?file=mar2012%2Fhe03132012_fee.pdf.

[65] Alaina Busch, "FDA Official: Guidance, Tracking Among Device Bills Clashing With Fee Pact," *InsideHealthPolicy.com*, March 28, 2012.

[66] Ibid.

[67] Ibid.

Appendix A. Provisions in FFDCA §737 and §738

Table A-1. Provisions in Section 737 and 738 of the Federal Food, Drug, and Cosmetic Act Relating to Medical Device User Fees

Main Issue	Current Law	MDUFA III Statutory Language that HHS Submitted to Congress
Section 737. Definitions.		
Definitions	Provides definitions for a number of terms.	Would update the definition of "adjustment factor" and change the definition of "establishment subject to a registration fee," increasing the number paying the fee from 16,000 to 22,000.
Section 738. Authority to Assess and Use Device Fees.		
(a)(1) Types of fees	There are several types of fees and certain exceptions to the collection of such fees.	
(a)(2)(A) PMA, premarket report, supplement, and submission fee, and annual fee for periodic reporting concerning a class III device	A fee is assessed for: premarket application (PMA) premarket report, equal to the PMA fee panel track supplement, 75% of the PMA fee 180-day supplement, 15% of the PMA fee real-time supplement, 7% of the PMA fee 30-day notice, 1.6% of the PMA fee efficacy supplement, equal to the PMA fee premarket notification submission [510(k)], 1.84% of the PMA fee request for classification information, 1.35% of the PMA fee periodic reporting concerning class III device, 3.5% of PMA fee.	Would set fee for 510(k) at 2% of the PMA fee
(a)(2)(B) Exceptions	Exceptions are made for humanitarian device exemption, PMA for a biologic product licensed for further manufacturing use only, devices sponsored by state or federal government and not intended for commercial distribution, 510(k) reviewed by an accredited third party, and PMAs, premarket reports and 510(k)s if the device is intended solely for a pediatric population, as well as supplements proposing conditions of use for a pediatric population.	
(a)(2)(C)(D) Payment, Refund	The fee is due at the time of submission. Partial or full refunds of fees either may or must occur, depending on certain conditions.	
(a)(3) Annual establishment registration fee	An establishment registration fee is assessed annually. Exceptions are made for an establishment operated by state or federal government entity, and Indian tribes unless the device is intended for commercial distribution.	Would make technical change to date payable.

Main Issue	Current Law	MDUFA III Statutory Language that HHS Submitted to Congress
(b) Fee amounts	Fees are based on the following amounts which may be adjusted by the Secretary for various reasons: PMA Estab ishment FY2008 $185,000 $1,706 FY2009 $200,725 $1,851 FY2010 $217,787 $2,008 FY2011 $236,298 $2,179 FY2012 $256,384 $2,364	New (b)(1)-(2). Would change fee amounts and change reasons for adjustment: PMA Establish. FY2013: $248,000; $2,575 FY2014: $252,960; $3,200 FY2015: $258,019; $3,750 FY2016: $263,180; $3,872 FY2017: $268,443; $3,872
(h) Crediting and availabi ity of fees	FY2008 $48,431,000 [FY2013 $95,429,314] FY2009 $52,547,000 [FY2014 $112,171,877] FY2010 $57,014,000 [FY2015 $127,537,959] FY2011 $61,860,000 [FY2016 $129,997,509] FY2012 $67,118,000 [FY2017 $130,328,967] Bracketed amounts in proposal, not current law.	Total revenue amounts, new (b)(3). Would set total fee revenue amounts as follows: FY2013 $97,722,301 FY2014 $112,580,497 FY2015 $125,767,107 FY2016 $129,339,949 FY2017 $130,184,348.
(c)(1) Annual fee setting; in general	The Secretary publishes fee amounts in the Federal Register 60 days before the start of each fiscal year.	Secretary would, 60 days before the start of each fiscal year, establish fees based on amounts specified in subsection (b) and the adjustments in this subsection, and pub ish such fees and rationale for adjusting fee amounts in the Federal Register.

Main Issue	Current Law	MDUFA III Statutory Language that HHS Submitted to Congress
(c)(2) Adjustment	The Secretary may increase the establishment fee for FY2010 only if the estimate of number of establishments submitting fees for FY2009 is less than 12,250. If the fee for FY2010 is adjusted, fees for FY2011 and FY2012 may be increased by 8.5% over the previous year. The determination and its rationale must be published in the Federal Register.	Inflation adjustment. Would adjust total revenue amounts by a specified inflation adjustment based on the sum of one plus—the average annual change in the cost per FTE position at FDA of all personnel compensation and benefits paid for the first 3 years of the preceding 4 fiscal years, multiplied by 0.60, and the average annual change in the Consumer Price Index (Metro DC, Baltimore, WV. not seasonally adjusted, all items, annual index) for the first 3 years of the preceding 4 years of available data multiplied by 0.40. If the sum is less than 1, the sum is considered to be 1; or greater than 1.04, the sum is considered to be 1.04. The base fee amounts in new subsection (b)(2) would be adjusted as needed on a uniform proportional basis to generate the inflation adjusted total revenue amount.
Adjustment to establishment registration base fees	No provision.	New (c)(3). For each fiscal year, after the base fee amounts in new subsection (b)(2) are adjusted for inflation, the base establishment registration fee amounts would be further adjusted as necessary for total fee collections for the fiscal year to generate the total adjusted revenue amount.
(c)(3) Limit	For each fiscal year, the total amount of fees, as adjusted, may not exceed the total costs for the resources allocated for the process for the review of device applications.	Now (c)(4)
(c)(4) Supplement	Secretary may use unobligated carryover balances from fees collected in previous years to ensure sufficient fee revenues are available, so long as there is a certain operating reserve. Not later than 14 days before using these funds, the Secretary must provide notice to House and Senate Appropriation Committees, Senate HELP and House Energy and Commerce Committees.	Now (c)(5)

Main Issue	Current Law	MDUFA III Statutory Language that HHS Submitted to Congress
(d)(e) Small businesses; fee waiver and fee reduction	Secretary may waive the fee for the first premarket review or first premarket report of a product submitted by a small business, defined as an entity that reported less than $30 million in gross receipts or sales in its most recent federal income tax return. If a device company has annual gross receipts or sales of $100 million or less in the most recent federal income tax return for a taxable year, including returns of its affiliates, the device manufacturer is a small business eligible for 75% reduction in fees for PMAs, premarket reports, supplements, and periodic reporting concerning class III devices. Such a device manufacturer is also considered a small business eigible for a reduced rate of 50% for fees regarding 510(k)s, 30-day notices and requests for classification information. Proof of gross sales or receipts may consist of IRS tax documents or qualifying documentation from the taxing authority of the foreign country in which the applicant or affi iate is headquartered.	
Fee waiver or reduction	No provision.	Would allow the Secretary to grant a waiver or reduced fees for a PMA or establishment fee if the waiver is in the interest of pub ic health. Waivers & fee reductions must be less than 2% of total fee revenue for that year. Authority for the waiver and reduced fees ends on October 1, 2017.
(f) Effect of failure to pay fees	PMAs, 510(k), requests for classification, and other submissions for which fees apply will not be accepted if fees are not paid.	
(g) Conditions (Trigger)	Direct appropriations must be more than 1% less than $205,720,000 multip ied by an adjustment factor, or else the Secretary may not collect user fees and is not required to meet performance goals.	Changes amount to $280,587,000.
(h) Crediting and availabi ity of fees	The following amounts of user fees are authorized to be appropriated: FY2008 $48,431,000 FY2009 $52,547,000 FY2010 $57,014,000 FY2011 $61,860,000 FY2012 $67,118,000 Offset is handled as follows: the amount of fees collected, in the first three fiscal years and estimated for the fourth fiscal year, in excess of the amount specified in appropriations acts is credited to FDA's appropriation account, and the excess subtracted from the amount that would otherwise have been authorized to be collected during the fifth fiscal year.	Would add provision allowing the Secretary to accept early payment of authorized fees. Would authorize to be appropriated for FY2013 through FY2017 fees equal to the total revenue amount as specified under new subsection(b)(3), as adjusted for inflation and offset.
(i) Collection of unpaid fees	Any unpaid fee shall be treated as a claim of the United States Government.	

Main Issue	Current Law	MDUFA III Statutory Language that HHS Submitted to Congress
(j) Written requests for refunds	A sponsor must submit a written request to the Secretary for a refund not later than 180 days after the fee is due.	
(k) Construction	"This section may not be construed to require that" HHS reduce FTE positions of officers, employees, and advisory committee members in other areas to offset those "engaged in the process of the review of device applications."	

Sources: FFDCA §§737-738 (21 U.S.C. §§379i-379j); and FDA, "Draft MDUFA III Legislative Language," dated February 17, 2012, posted on FDA website March 14, 2012, at http://www.fda.gov/downloads/MedicalDevices/NewsEvents/WorkshopsConferences/UCM295424.pdf.

Note: Paragraph and subparagraph labeing follows current law.

Table A-2. Provisions in Draft MDUFA III Legislative Language That Would Add Two New Sections to Chapter VII of the Federal Food, Drug, and Cosmetic Act

Main Issue	Provision Included in Draft MDUFA Legislation
Subchapter D—Information and Education Section 74x	Would require that after final guidance is issued, PMA, 510(k), Product Development Protocol, Investigational Device Exemption (IDE), Humanitarian Device Exemption (HDE), and other specified pre- submissions and submissions, and any supplements to such submissions must include an electronic copy.
Subchapter A—General Administrative Provisions Section 7xx Stream ined hiring authority	Would allow the Secretary, without regard to provisions in title 5 U.S.C., to appoint employees to appoint FDA employees to positions related to the process for the review of device applications in order to achieve the performance goals referred to in section 738A(a)(1) as set forth in the Secretary's Commitment Letter. The authority to appoint such employees would terminate three years after the date of enactment.

Source: FDA, "Draft MDUFA III Legislative Language," dated February 17, 2012, posted on FDA website March 14, 2012, at http://www.fda.gov/downloads/MedicalDevices/NewsEvents/WorkshopsConferences/UCM295424.pdf.

Appendix B. MDUFA III Agreement: Performance Goals and Procedures

Table B-1. Performance Goals and Procedures in Agreement Between FDA and Industry Representatives for FY2013 through FY2017 Under the Draft MDUFA III

Topic	Draft MDUFA III commitments	Similar language in MDUFA II commitments
I. Process Improvements	Pre-Submissions. FDA will issue draft guidance and final guidance on a new structured process for managing Pre-Submissions. Upon receipt of a Pre-Submission, FDA intends to schedule a one hour meeting or teleconference, if requested. Within 14 days of receipt, FDA will determine if the Pre-Submission meets the definition and notify the applicant if it does not. Three business days prior to meeting, FDA will provide initial feedback via email. FDA and app icant may cancel meeting if no longer needed based on email that will serve as final written feedback. Within 15 days, app icant provides draft minutes including agreements and action items, and FDA edits minutes which become final 15 days after received by app icant. FDA feedback is intended to be final, unless FDA concludes that the feedback does not address important new safety and effectiveness issues.	FDA will make every effort to schedule both informal and formal meetings, both before and during the review process, in a timely manner. These meetings include pre-submission meetings.
	Submission Acceptance Criteria. Prior to implementation, FDA will pub ish draft and final guidance on electronic submissions and objective criteria for revised "refuse to accept/refuse to file" check ists.	New section.
	Interactive Review. As described in current guidance, FDA will continue to use interactive review to encourage informal communication between agency and applicant to facilitate timely completion of the review process.	FDA will continue to use interactive review process to encourage communication and faci itate review.
	Guidance Document Development. FDA will apply user fees to the guidance document development process, but not to the detriment of meeting the quantitative review time ines and statutory ob igations. FDA will update its website, deleting outdated guidance, noting which are under review, and providing a ist of prioritized device guidance documents intended to be published within 12 months and other device guidance documents intended to be pub ished as resources permit.	FDA will develop guidance documents to the extent possible without impacting device review time and will post guidance under development for comment.
	Third Party Review. FDA will work with interested parties to improve the current program and transparency, but not to the detriment of meeting the quantitative review time ines and statutory ob igations.	
	Patient Safety and Risk Tolerance. FDA will fully implement final guidance on factors to consider when making benefit-risk determinations in device premarket review, including patient tolerance for risk, magnitude of benefit, and availability of other treatments or diagnostic tests.	New section.
	Low Risk Medical Device Exemptions. By the end of FY2013, FDA will propose additional low risk medical devices to exempt from the 510(k) process and intends to issue a final rule within 2 years exempting additional low risk devices from 510(k).	New section.

Topic	Draft MDUFA III commitments	Similar language in MDUFA II commitments
	Emerging Diagnostics. FDA will work with industry to develop a transitional in vitro diagnostics (IVD) approach for the regulation of emerging diagnostics.	To facilitate IVD development, FDA will explore ways to clarify the regulatory requirements by issuing guidance as well as 5 other specified activities.
II. Review performance goals	PMA, Panel-Track Supplements, and Premarket Report App ications. Performance goals apply to all PMAs, Panel-Track Supplements, and Premarket Report Applications including those that are priority review (previously referred to as expedited). FDA will communicate with applicant on status of app ication within 15 days of receipt. For submissions that do not require Advisory Committee input, FDA will issue a MDUFA decision within 180 FDA Days for: 70% of submissions received in FY2013; 80% of submissions received in FY2014 and FY2015; and 90% of submissions received in FY2016 and FY2017. For submissions that require Advisory Committee input, FDA will issue a MDUFA decision within 320 FDA Days for: 50% of submissions received in FY2013; 70% of submissions received in FY2014; 80% of submissions received in FY2015 and FY2016; and 90% of submissions received in FY2017. For all PMAs that do not reach a MDUFA decision by 20 days after the FDA Day goal, FDA will provide written feedback to the applicant including all outstanding issues preventing FDA from reaching a decision.	FDA will issue a decision for 60% of non-expedited filed submissions within 180 days, and for 90% within 295 days. FDA will issue a decision for 50% of expedited filed submissions within 180 days and for 90% within 280 days.
	180-Day PMA Supplements. FDA will communicate with applicant within 90 days of receipt of the submission for: 65% of submissions received in FY2013; 75% of submissions received in FY2014; 85% of submissions received in FY2015; and 95% of submissions received in FY2016 through FY2017. FDA will issue a MDUFA decision within 180 FDA Days for: 85% of submissions received in FY2013; 90% of submissions received in FY2014 and FY2015; and 95% of submissions received in FY2016 through FY2017.	FDA will issue a decision for 85% within 180 days and for 95% within 210 days.
	Real-Time PMA Supplements. FDA will issue a MDUFA decision within 90 FDA Days for: 90% of such submissions received in FY2013 and FY2014; and 95% of such submissions received in FY2015 through FY2017.	FDA will issue a decision for 80% within 60 days, and for 90% within 90 days.
	510(k) Submissions. FDA will communicate with applicant on status of application within 15 days of receipt. For submissions received in FY2013, FDA will issue a MDUFA decision for 91% of 510(k) submissions within 90 FDA Days. For submissions received in FY2014, FDA will issue a MDUFA decision for 93% of 510(k) submissions within 90 FDA Days. For submissions received in FY2015 through FY2017, FDA will issue a MDUFA decision for 95% of 510(k) submissions within 90 FDA Days. For all 510(k)s that do not reach a MDUFA decision within 100 FDA Days, FDA will provide written feedback to the applicant including all outstanding issues preventing FDA from reaching a decision.	FDA will issue a decision for 90% of 510(k)s within 90 days, and for 98% within 150 days.

Topic	Draft **MDUFA III** commitments	Similar language in **MDUFA II** commitments
	CLIA Waiver by Application. During the pre-submission process, if the applicant informs FDA that it plans to submit a dual submission (510(k) and CLIA Waiver application), FDA will issue a decision for 90% of such applications within 210 FDA days. For "CLIA Waiver by Application" submissions FDA will issue a MDUFA decision: for 95% of the applications that do not require Advisory Committee input within 180 FDA days; for 95% of the applications that require Advisory Committee input within 330 FDA days. FDA will issue guidance regarding review and management expectations to provide greater transparency throughout the entire submission process.	New section.
	Biologics Licensing Applications (BLAs). FDA will review and act on standard original BLA submissions within 10 months of receipt for 90% of submissions. FDA will review and act on priority original BLA submissions within 6 months of receipt for 90% of submissions. FDA will review and act on standard BLA efficacy supplement submissions within 10 months of receipt for 90% of submissions. FDA will review and act on priority BLA efficacy supplement submissions within 6 months of receipt for 90% of submissions. FDA will review and act on Class 1 original BLA and BLA efficacy supplement resubmissions within 2 months of receipt for 90% of submissions. FDA will review and act on Class 2 original BLA and BLA efficacy supplement resubmissions within 6 months of receipt for 90% of submissions. FDA will review and act on BLA manufacturing supplements requiring prior approval within 4 months of receipt for 90% of submissions.	90% of BLAs in 10 months. 90% of BLA supplements in 10 months. 90% of BLA resubmissions and BLA supplement resubmissions in two months
III. Shared Outcome Goal	Process improvements in the agreement are intended to reduce the average Total Time to Decision for PMAs and 510(k)s. FDA and applicants share the responsibility for achieving this goal.	New section.
	PMA. For submissions received beginning in FY2013, the average Total Time to Decision goal for FDA and industry is 395 calendar days; beginning in FY2015, 390 calendar days; beginning in FY2017, 385 calendar days.	
	510(k). For submissions received beginning in FY2013, the average Total Time to Decision goal for FDA and industry is 135 calendar days; beginning in FY2015, 130 calendar days; beginning in FY2017, 124 calendar days.	
IV. Infrastructure	Scientific and Regulatory Review Capacity. User fees will be used to reduce the ratio of review staff to supervisors and to enhance and supplement scientific review capacity by hiring reviewers and leveraging external experts needed to assist with device application review. FDA will seek to obtain streamlined hiring authority and work with industry to benchmark best practices for retaining employees (both financial and non-financial).	New section.
	Training. FDA will hold at least two medical device Vendor Days each year. User fees will supplement the following: management training; MDUFA III train for all staff; Reviewer Certification Program for new reviewers; specialized training to provide continuous learning for all staff.	FDA will apply user fees to support reviewer training that is related to the process for the review of devices, including training to enhance scientific expertise.

Topic	Draft MDUFA III commitments	Similar language in MDUFA II commitments
	Tracking System. IT system will be improved to allow real-time status information for submissions.	New section.
V. Independent Assessment of Review Process Management	By the end of the 2nd quarter of FY2013, FDA will award a contract to assess the device application review process. Within 6 months of award, a report on recommendations likely to have a significant impact on review time will be published; final report will be published within 1 year of contract award. FDA will publish an implementation plan within 6 months of receipt of each report. The contractor will evaluate FDA's implementation and publish a report no later than February 1, 2016.	New section.
VI. Performance Reports	Information to be covered in quarterly reports by CDRH and CBER is isted for: 510(k)s, PMAs; Pre-Submissions; and, IDEs. CDRH reports quarterly and CBER reports annually on 11 data points such as: NSE decisions for 510(k)s; withdrawls of 510(k)s and PMAs; not approvable decisions for PMAs; other noteworthy issues ike rates of AI letters; number of submissions that missed goals; new draft and final guidance; fee collection summary; independent assessment implementation plan status; number of discretionary fee waivers. FDA reports annually on nine topics such as: use of fees for enhanced scientific review capacity; number of Premarket Report Submissions; summary of training courses; shared outcome goal performance; 510(k) submissions; PMA submissions; DeNovo classification petitions; CLIA waiver app ications.	FDA reports quarterly on progress toward attaining quantitative goals. For all submission types, FDA will track total time from receipt to final decision. FDA provides annually review performance data by branch (grouped by subject), indicating the shortest and longest average review times for 510(k)s, 180-day supplements, and real-time supplements.
VII. Discretionary Waiver	FDA will seek authority to grant discretionary fee waivers or reduced fees in the interest of pub ic health. Authority for the waiver and reduced fees expires at the end of MDUFA III.	New section.
VIII. Definitions and explanations of terms	Total Time to Decision is the number of calendar days from the date to receipt or filed submission to a MDUFA decision. The average Total Time to Decision for 510(k) submissions is calculated as the trimmed mean of Total Times to Decision for 510(k) submissions within a closed cohort, excluding the highest 2% and the lowest 2% of values. A cohort is closed when 99% of the accepted submissions have reached a decision. A cohort consists of all submissions of a certain type, in this case 510(k), filed in the same fiscal year. The average Total Time to Decision for PMA applications is calculated as the three-year rolling average of the annual Total Times to Decision for applications (for example, for FY2015, the average Total Time to Decision for PMA applications would be the average of FY2013 through FY2015) within a closed cohort, excluding the highest 5% and the lowest 5% of values. A cohort is closed when 95% of the applications have reached a decision. A cohort consists of all submissions of a certain type, in this case PMA, filed in the same fiscal year. Other terms that are defined: App icant; Electronic Copy; FDA Days; MDUFA decisions; Pre-Submission; and, Substantive Interaction. Three BLA-related definitions are also provided: Review and act on; Class 1 resubmitted applications; and, Class 2 resubmitted applications.	The following terms were defined: FDA Decision; Expedited Review; PMA Modules; 180-Day PMA Supplements; and, Real-Time Supplements.

Source: FDA, "Draft MDUFA III Commitment Letter," dated February 17, 2012, and posted on FDA website March 14, 2012, at http://www.fda.gov/downloads/MedicalDevices/NewsEvents/WorkshopsConferences/

UCM295454.pdf. Document is referred to, at times, as the Commitment Letter or the Agreement; and FDA, "MDUFA 2007 Commitment Letter," dated September 27, 2007, and posted on FDA website at http://www.fda.gov/MedicalDevices/DeviceRegulationandGuidance/Overview/ MedicalDeviceUserFeeandModernizationActMDUFMA/default.htm.

Note: Topic numbering corresponds to the ordering in draft MDUFA III Agreement; these are usually different from the MDUFA II (2007) numbering.

Appendix C. MDUFMA and MDUFA: Fees and Performance Goals

Table C-1. MDUFMA/MDUFA 2007 Fee Schedule, FY2007-FY2012

	MDUFMA	MDUFA 2007				
Fees Structure	**2007**	**2008**	**2009**	**2010**	**2011**	**2012**
Application Fees						
PMA (i.e., *base fee*)	$281,600	$185,000	$200,725	$217,787	$236,298	$256,384
Small Business[a]	$107,008	$46,250	$50,181	$54,447	$59,075	$64,096
Panel Track Supplement[b]	$281,600	$138,750	$150,544	$163,340	$177,224	$192,288
Small Business[a]	$107,008	$34,688	$37,636	$40,835	$44,306	$48,072
180-Day Supplement[c]	$60,544	$27,750	$30,109	$32,668	$35,445	$38,458
Small Business[a]	$23,007	$6,938	$7,527	$8,167	$8,861	$9,614
Real Time Supplement[d]	$20,275	$12,950	$14,051	$15,245	$16,541	$17,947
Small Business[a]	$7,705	$3,237	$3,512	$3,810	$4,134	$4,485
510(k)	$4,158	$3,404	$3,693	$4,007	$4,348	$4,717
Small Business[a]	$3,326	$1,702	$1,847	$2,004	$2,174	$2,359
30-Day Notice[e]		$2,960	$3,212	$3,485	$3,781	$4,102
Small Business[a]		$1,480	$1,606	$1,742	$1,890	$2,051
513(g)[f]		$2,498	$2,710	$2,940	$3,190	$3,461
Small Business[a]		$1,249	$1,355	$1,470	$1,595	$1,731
Product Fee						
Annual Fee for Periodic Report.		$6,475	$7,025	$7,623	$8,270	$8,973
Small Business[a]		$1,619	$1,756	$1,906	$2,068	$2,243
Establishment Fee						
Establishment Registration		$1,706	$1,851	$2,008	$2,179	$2,364

Source: FDA, *Medical Devices: Proposed Industry User Fee Schedule for MDUFMA II*, March 3, 2009, accessed on January 31, 2012, http://www.fda.gov/MedicalDevices/DeviceRegulationandGuidance/Overview/MedicalDeviceUserFeeandModernizationActMDUFMA/ucm109319.htm.

a. Small Business—indicates the reduced small business fee associated with the item isted above.

b. Panel-Track Supplement—manufacturer requests approval of a significant change in the design or performance of a device approved via the PMA pathway; significant amount of clinical data evaluated.

c. 180-Day PMA Supplement—manufacturer requests approval of a change in aspects of an approved device, such as its design, specifications, or labeling; new clinical data not required or only limited c inical data.

d. Real-Time PMA Supplement—manufacturer requests approval for a minor change to an approved device, such as a minor change in the design or labeling.

e. 30-Day Notice—manufacturer requests permission to make modifications to manufacturing procedures or methods of manufacture affecting the safety and effectiveness of the device.

f. 513(g)—manufacturer requests information on the classification of a device.

Appendix D. MDUFA III Performance Goals

Table D-1. Summary of Performance Goals per February 7, 2012, Agreement

Submission Type		2007	2008-2012	2013-2017 (01/31/2012 Agreement) - all in FDA Days except Average Total				
		End of MDUFMA I	MDUFA II	FY13	FY14	FY15	FY16	FY17
510(k)	Tier 1	80% in 90 days	90% in 90 days	91% in 90 days	93% in 90 days	95% in 90 days	95% in 90 days	95% in 90 days
	Tier 2	N.A.	98% in 150 days					
	Cycle	90% in 75 days	N.A.	N.A.	N.A.	N.A.	N.A.	N.A.
	Interaction	N.A.	N.A.	65% in 60 days	75% in 60 days	85% in 60 days	95% in 60 days	95% in 60 days
	Average Total Time	N.A.	N.A.	135 days	135 days	130 days	130 days	124 days
180 Day PMA Supplement	Tier 1	90% in 180 days	85% in 180 days	85% in 180 days	90% in 180 days	90% in 180 days	95% in 180 days	95% in 180 days
	Tier 2	N.A.	95% in 210 days					
	Cycle	90% in 120 days	N.A.	N.A.	N.A.	N.A.	N.A.	N.A.
	Interaction	N.A.	N.A.	65% in 90 days	75% in 90 days	85% in 90 days	95% in 90 days	95% in 90 days
Original PMAs & Panel Track Supplements		Tier 1 - 50% in 180 days	Tier 1 - 60% in 180 days	No Panel - 70% in 180 days	No Panel - 80% in 180 days	No Panel - 80% in 180 days	No Panel - 90% in 180 days	No Panel - 90% in 180 days
		Tier 2 - 90% in 320 days	Tier 2 - 90% in 295 days	With Panel - 50% in 320 days	With Panel - 70% in 320 days	With Panel - 80% in 320 days	With Panel - 80% in 320 days	With Panel - 90% in 320 days
	Cycle	75% in 150 days	N.A.	N.A.	N.A.	N.A.	N.A.	N.A.
	Interaction	N.A.	N.A.	65% in 90 days	75% in 90 days	85% in 90 days	95% in 90 days	95% in 90 days
	Average Total Time	N.A.	N.A.	395 days	395 days	390 days	390 days	385 days
Expedited PMAs	Tier 1	90% in 300 days	50% in 180 days	Included with "Original PMAs"	Included with "Original PMAs"	Included with "Original PMAs"	Included with "Original PMAs"	Included with "Original PMAs"
	Tier 2	N.A.	90% in 280 days					
	Cycle	70% in 120 days	N.A.	90% in 90 days	90% in 90 days	95% in 90 days	95% in 90 days	95% in 90 days
Real Time PMA Supplements	Tier 1	N.A.	80% in 60 days	90% in 210 days	95% in 180 days	95% in 180 days	95% in 180 days	90% in 90 days
	Tier 2	N.A.	90% in 90 days	90% in 180 days	95% in 330 days	95% in 330 days	95% in 330 days	95% in 330 days

Submission Type		2007	2008-2012	2013-2017 (01/31/2012 Agreement) - all in FDA Days except Average Total				
		End of MDUFMA I	MDUFA II	FY13	FY14	FY15	FY16	FY17
CLIA Waiver Applications	Dual CLIA/ 510(k)	N.A.	N.A.	90% in 210 days	90% in 210 days	90% in 210 days	90% in 210 days	90% in 210 days
	CLIA – no panel	N.A.	N.A.	95% in 180 days	95% in 180 days	95% in 180 days	95% in 180 days	95% in 180 days
	CLIA – with panel	N.A.	N.A.	95% in 330 days	95% in 330 days	95% in 330 days	95% in 330 days	95% in 330 days

Source: FDA, MDUFA Reauthorization Public Meeting, Slide 17, March 28, 2012.

Note: N.A. = Not App icable.

Appendix E. Acronyms Used in This Report

510(k)	Premarket Notification
513(g)	Request for Information About Device Classification
BLA	Biologics License Application
CBER	Center for Biologics Evaluation and Research
CDRH	Center for Devices and Radiological Health
CLIA	Clinical Laboratory Improvement Amendments
FDA	United States Food and Drug Administration
FFDCA	Federal Food, Drug, and Cosmetic Act (21 U.S.C. Chapter 9)
FTE	Full Time Equivalent Employee
GAO	Government Accountability Office (formerly General Accounting Office)
HDE	Humanitarian Device Exemption
HELP	Senate Health, Education, Labor and Pensions Committee
HHS	United States Department of Health and Human Services
IDE	Investigational Device Exemption
MDTCA	Medical Device Technical Corrections Act
MDUFMA	Medical Device User Fee and Modernization Act
MDUFA II	Medical Device User Fee Amendments of 2007
MDUFSA	Medical Device User Fee Stabilization Act of 2005
MQSA	Mammography Quality Standards Act
NSE	Non-Substantial Equivalence
PDP	Product Development Protocol
PDUFA	Prescription Drug User Fee Act
PL	Public Law
PMA	Premarket Approval
RIF	Reduction in Force
SE	Substantial Equivalence
SUD	Single-Use Device
USC	United States Code

Author Contact Information

Judith A. Johnson
Specialist in Biomedical Policy
jajohnson@crs.loc.gov, 7-7077

MY DEVELOPMENT COMMITMENT

Conforming: Dimming Star

You are demonstrating declining performance outcomes and/or declining passionate behaviors or attitude toward the work, colleagues or manager. Is the work not challenging or is the work lacking personal meaning? Has there been a change in leadership, manager, or a significant life event?

Reignite the Passion-Performance with Meaning

- **Conduct a work environment scan** to assess resources, time pressures or organizational changes that may be out of your control.
- **Assess life-work factors** and impact on passion decline.
- **Listen to others' perspectives** on your work attitude.
- **Assess career aspirations** and unfulfilled dreams.
- **Assess reward alignment** with your primary passion and lifestyle motivators.
- **Assess emerging or declining interests** and task "misfits."
- **Assess interpersonal needs** of inclusion, control and performance feedback.
- **Conduct feedback** to identify hidden strengths—or blind spots.
- **Consider career options** to explore new opportunities, enrich current job or movement to a new job or career.

Storming: Fallen Star

Time to conduct a reality check about your work attitude. Seek feedback on how others (manager, peer, customers, friends) perceive your strengths and the value you bring to the business. It is time to assess and realign your natural talents and passions with performance tasks.

Rediscover Potential—Determine the BestFit

- **Time to reality check** your work attitude.
- **Invest in a BestFit Career Alignment Assessment.**
- **Seek feedback** on your skill strengths and core competency from peers, customers and and manager.
- **Explore perception gaps** (hidden strengths and blind spots).
- **Seek new or previous performance tasks** or projects that optimize core talents.
- **Determine the impact** of the work or leadership climate on your declining passion or performance.
- **Seek coaching** on emotional intelligence or career skills.
- **Be clear on your role** in directing change.
- **Be clear on consequences** of doing nothing.
- **Seek to understand why you *delay* in moving forward**—is it fear of success or failure?
- **Ask for coaching sessions** with clear progress indicators.

WORKPLACE COACH
INSTITUTE

Smart2Smarter by Kivland, 2011 (www.smart2smarter.com)
For exclusive one time use by the Smart2Smarter Community and participants
in Social and Emotional Intelligence Coach or Leader Certification Program,
Workplace Coach Institute, © 2003-2010 Cynthia Kivland, President
For group distribution or reproduction costs, contact cynthia@Smart2Smarter.com

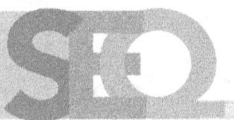
 SMARTER REFLECTIONS

Use this space to record your SMARTER thoughts, reflections, actions and goals.

Smart2Smarter by Kivland, 2011 (www.smart2smarter.com)
For exclusive one time use by the Smart2Smarter Community and participants
in Social and Emotional Intelligence Coach or Leader Certification Program,
Workplace Coach Institute, © 2003-2010 Cynthia Kivland, President
For group distribution or reproduction costs, contact cynthia@Smart2Smarter.com

Chapter 4 Strengths

Workplace Engagement Values

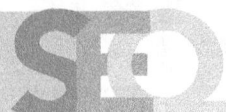
Join the *Smart 2 Smarter Community*
to ENGAGE SMARTER

WORKPLACE COACH
I N S T I T U T E inc

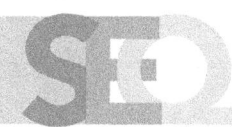
WORKPLACE ENGAGEMENT AND PASSION

Do you feel fully or somewhat engaged in your current job? Do you feel you are contributing your personal best, or do you feel you would be better off somewhere else? If you answered yes to the latter part of the question, can you define what better off means for you?

The following Workplace Engagement Values Assessment will help you establish what needs to be present in order for you to fully engage in a job activity.

Workplace engagement values are what drives the passion a person brings to his or her work. Passion is the natural energy, motivation and enthusiasm about how you contribute in the world of work. Workplace Engagement or "FLOW" is being energized, focused, positive, blissful and absorbed in the activity in a seemingly effortless and fluid way.

When a workplace engagement value is satisfied, an individual is fully engaged to contribute their *personal best*. When absent or neglected, the engagement fuel and spark are missing. For example, believing in the value of the subject they are teaching often sparks the commitment and energy teachers bring to their work.

To sum up, a great way to clarify what fosters and engages your work FLOW is to understand what you value. Your values are the foundation of a career development plan, helping you identify the job satisfiers you want, and often need, to contribute your personal best.

Workplace engagement values can be divided into two categories: Intrinsic and Extrinsic.

INTRINSIC values relate to a specific interest in the work activity or the benefit of the work to society.

EXTRINSIC values relate to the preferred conditions of an occupational choice, such as physical setting, earning potential or benefits.

However, research indicates that meeting your intrinsic values results in increased work satisfaction, motivation and engagement.

The BestFit Career Star
PassionFit

PurposeFit   PerformanceFit

ProfessionFit   PeopleFit

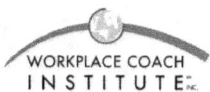
Smart2Smarter by Kivland, 2011 (www.smart2smarter.com)
For exclusive one time use by the Smart2Smarter Community and participants
in Social and Emotional Intelligence Coach or Leader Certification Program,
Workplace Coach Institute, © 2003-2010 Cynthia Kivland, President
For group distribution or reproduction costs, contact cynthia@Smart2Smarter.com

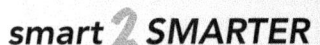 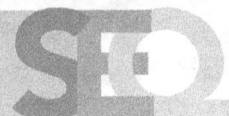
 WHAT DEFINES A VALUE?

Criteria help to better assess what values drive your life and work decisions. Use three criteria when you answer the value statements. These three criteria are: 1) Choosing, 2) Prizing, and 3) Acting.

Criterion One CHOOSING

- I choose the value freely, without pressure from other people or society.

- I choose the value from other alternatives or choices.

- I choose the value after thoughtful consideration of the consequences of each choice.

Criterion Two PRIZING

- I prize and cherish my values. My values define who I am and I cherish what I do.

- I publicly affirm my values. I have chosen this value freely, after consideration of the consequences, therefore I inform others about it when appropriate.

Criterion Three ACTING

- I act on my values. The value means something to me; therefore I commit time and energy to the value.

- I act on the value repeatedly. I do not act on the value just once but the value is a life habit.

When you examine your values, you are also looking at how the role of work currently fits in your life.
Your values may not be the same at twenty, thirty or fifty years old. It is important to assess your values annually as what you want (value) from your work may, and often does, change.

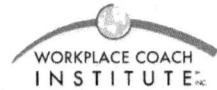

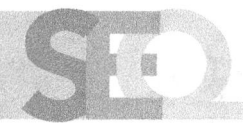
 WORKPLACE ENGAGEMENT VALUES ASSESSMENT INSTRUCTIONS

Directions

On page 14, there are ten pairs of statements describing value choices concerning your preferred work environment.

Step 1 For each pair of statements, choose the statement that best describes you and put an "**(x)**" next to the statement in Column A. *Example:*

#	Statement	A	High Engagement (FLOW)	Moderate Engagement	Some Engagement
1	I prefer to work alone or as an individual contributor.	X			
	I prefer to work with others and be associated with the team or organization.				

Step 2 Put an "**(x)**" in the column if the Value Statement inspires *High Work Engagement (FLOW), Moderate Engagement* or *Some Engagement* in the job or task activity. *Example:*

#	Statement	A	High Engagement (FLOW)	Moderate Engagement	Some Engagement
1	I prefer to work alone or as an individual contributor.	X		X	
	I prefer to work with others and be associated with the team or organization.				

Step 3 Next you will see which values you have checked. For each value you have chosen, mark appropriately if it is/was present or absent at your current/past job.

#	Statement	A	High Engagement (FLOW)	Moderate Engagement	Some Engagement	Present at work	Absent at work
1	I prefer to work alone or as an individual contributor. Independence.	X		X		X	
	I prefer to work with others and be associated with the team or organization. Affiliation.						

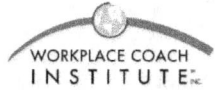
Smart2Smarter by Kivland, 2011 (www.smart2smarter.com)
For exclusive one time use by the Smart2Smarter Community and participants
in Social and Emotional Intelligence Coach or Leader Certification Program.
Workplace Coach Institute, © 2003-2010 Cynthia Kivland, President
For group distribution or reproduction costs, contact cynthia@Smart2Smarter.com

Workplace Engagement Values
Chapter Four - Resource Tool

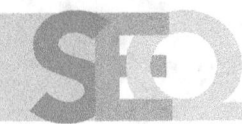
 WORKPLACE ENGAGEMENT VALUES ASSESSMENT

#	Statement	A	HIgh	Moderate	Some	Present at work	Absent at work
1	I prefer to work alone or as an individual contributor. **Independence.**						
	I prefer to work with others and be associated with the team or organization. **Affiliation.**						
2	I prefer to be in charge or in a position of authority. **Authority.**						
	I prefer to be regarded as a subject matter expert. **Expertise.**						
3	I prefer a secure work environment or profession and steady salary. **Security.**						
	I prefer an entrepreneurial work environment and open salary. **Entrepreneurship.**						
4	I prefer to take risks to obtain a "better fit" position seeking start-ups or new ventures. **Risktaking.**						
	I prefer not to take risks and seek stable occupations or companies. **Stability.**						
5	I prefer a set work schedule and routine. **Time Schedule.**						
	I prefer to set my own work schedule as long as the work gets done. **Time Freedom.**						
6	I prefer to compete with others in the work environment. **Competition.**						
	I prefer to work in a team where no one stands out. **Collaboration.**						
7	High-income potential or material gain is my primary motivator. **Materialism.**						
	Meaningful work is my primary motivator. **Altruism.**						
8	I prefer formal organizations with set rules, job descriptions and procedures. **Formal Environment.**						
	I prefer organizations with an informal, flexible work environment. **Informal Environment.**						
9	It is important to be in a profession/company that offers training for career and personal growth. **Personal Growth.**						
	It is important to be in a profession/company that offers training for job performance only. **Peformance Growth.**						
10	I prefer a position that directly involves working with people. **People Focus.**						
	I prefer a position that involves working with data, ideas or things. **Data, Things or Ideas Focus.**						

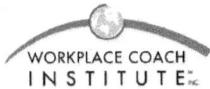

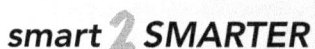
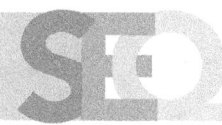
 UNDERSTANDING MY WORKPLACE ENGAGEMENT VALUES

My Workplace Engagement Values

Step 4 In the table below, write the top three values (from the columns *High Engagement*/*FLOW* and *Moderate Engagement*) that are *present* at your current/past job in the left column, and those that are *absent* in the right column.

My top three Workplace Engagement Values that are *Present*	My top three Workplace Engagement Values that are *Absent*
1.	1.
2.	2.
3.	3.

Reflection Activity

- What do your values say about what you need to stay engaged to contribute your personal best?

- What do your values tell you about how you define being successful?

- How do your values match with your organization's core values?

- Refer to those top values that you marked as high engagement/moderate engagement and which are/were fulfilled at your current/past job. How does that affect your career satisfaction and performance results?

- Refer to those top values that you have marked as high engagement/moderate engagement and which are/were not fulfilled at your current/past job. How does/did that affect your career satisfaction and performance results?

- Imagine choosing a career or job where your top values are not present. How does that feel?

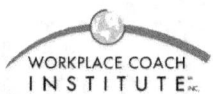 WORKPLACE COACH INSTITUTE INC.

Smart2Smarter by Kivland, 2011 (www.smart2smarter.com)
For exclusive one time use by the Smart2Smarter Community and participants
in Social and Emotional Intelligence Coach or Leader Certification Program.
Workplace Coach Institute, © 2003-2010 Cynthia Kivland, President
For group distribution or reproduction costs, contact cynthia@Smart2Smarter.com

Workplace Engagement Values
Chapter Four - Resource Tool

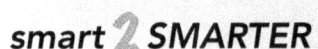 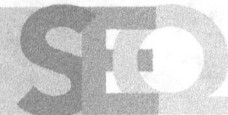

 UNDERSTANDING MY WORKPLACE ENGAGEMENT VALUES

Value Statement Activity

Step 5 Using the top values you selected as *High Engagement/FLOW* and *Moderate Engagement*, create a specific "What I value" statement.

Example:
I value consistent work hours; I want to work Monday through Friday from 9:00 p.m. until 5:00 p.m. This is important to me so I can be home with my family.

Statement 1

Statement 2

Statement 3

Statement 4

Statement 5

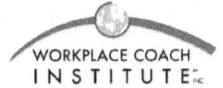

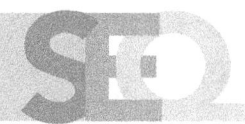
 ## WORKPLACE ENGAGEMENT VALUES ACTION PLAN

Step 6 Refer to the values that must be present to fully engage you in your career and prepare a Forward Action Plan.

1. What can you do on a daily basis that will keep your top values a priority?

2. How will others (family, spouse/partner, peers, boss) know that these values are your priority?

Who	How they will know

3. How can others (family, spouse/partner, peers, boss) support you in keeping these values a priority?

Who	What they can do

4. What do you need to stop tolerating (beliefs, excuses, behaviors) that prevents some of your values from becoming a priority?

What beliefs?	How to manage better
What excuses?	**How to manage better**
What behaviors?	**How to manage better**

WORKPLACE COACH
INSTITUTE inc.

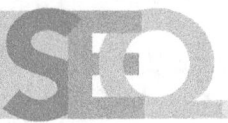
 SMARTER REFLECTIONS

Use this space to record your SMARTER thoughts, reflections, actions and goals.

Join the SMARTER Community
to Bring Humanity and Civility Back Into the Workplace!

What will you find on Smart2Smarter.com?

- Over 100 social and emotional intelligence tools

- Daily skill-building workouts

- Downloadable coaching activities and articles

- SMARTER career nuggets for smart people and leaders

- Workplace training and coach certification programs on leadership, resilience, career direction, emotional intelligence, empathy and more

- Seamless online ordering

- Guidelines and information on how to become a *Smart2Smarter* affiliate

- Global community of authors, researchers, consultants and coaches

This is the first website dedicated to bringing humanity and civility back into the workplace...

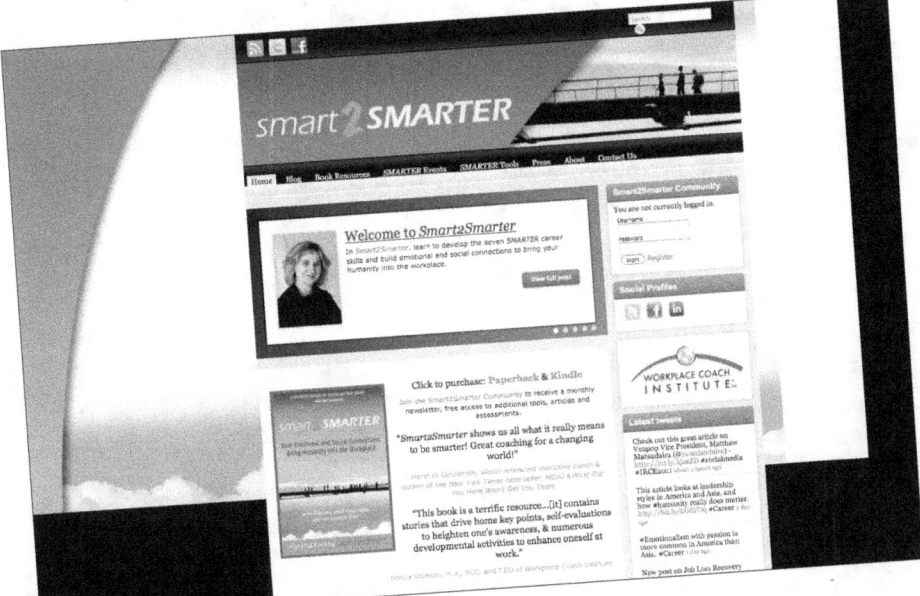

To inquire about having Cynthia speak at your next conference, workplace or special event, contact: Cynthia@Smart2Smarter.com

www.ingramcontent.com/pod-product-compliance
Lightning Source LLC
Chambersburg PA
CBHW081420170526
45166CB00010B/3422